THE DOCTOR'S BEAUTY HOTLINE

THE
DOCTOR'S
BEAUTY
HOTLINE

Dr. Fredric Haberman
   and
Margaret Danbrot

Illustrations by Judy Francis

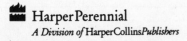
HarperPerennial
A Division of HarperCollins*Publishers*

NOTE

This book contains recommendations to be followed within the context of an overall health-care program. However, not all recommendations are designed for all individuals. While the book discusses certain issues and choices regarding skin care, it is not intended as a substitute for professional medical advice. Before following these or any other health-care recommendations, a physician should be consulted.

In applying and using drugs and cosmetics, consumers should follow the specific instructions provided by manufacturers. In addition, where drugs and pharmaceutical products are available only by prescription, users should always be sure to continue to consult with their dermatologists or medical specialists during the entire course of any treatment.

A hardcover edition of this book was published in 1990 by Henry Holt and Company. It is here reprinted by arrangement with Henry Holt and Company.

First HarperPerennial edition published 1991.

LIBRARY OF CONGRESS CATALOG CARD NUMBER 90-55975
ISBN 0-06-097391-9

91 92 93 94 95 MB 10 9 8 7 6 5 4 3 2 1

To my father, Harvey H. Haberman, and to the loving memory of my mother, Sylvia Haberman, and my cousin and dear friend, Roy Lester. And of course to Sheila, Renée, and Elisa, who always see me through.

Contents

Acknowledgments

I want to acknowledge with thanks and much appreciation Channa Taub, my editor, for her hard work, patience, and invaluable help at every stage of the manuscript, and my agent, Connie Clausen, for her friendly support and advice.

Susan Allen and the rest of my terrific office staff offered assistance above and beyond throughout the writing of this book, and Barbara Pipines provided much valuable insight. Thank you all.

My gratitude, too, to Michael Fisher, M.D., my chief of dermatology at Montefiore Medical Center/Albert Einstein College of Medicine, who remains an example, and to my colleagues at the American Medical Association Health Reporting Conference for their commitment to ethical, accurate, and clear health reporting.

And very special thanks to my patients for sharing the concerns that inspired this book.

F.H.

Introduction

A *doctor* writing a *beauty* book? A few words of explanation may be in order here.

Not long ago it occurred to me that as a dermatologist I sometimes spend almost as much time giving out beauty information as I do medical advice. It's not that my patients are more concerned with their looks than with their health. It's just that when someone comes to my office with a medical condition, he or she is apt to ask a few questions about less serious problems that affect the appearance.

For example, after assuring one of my patients that the mole she was worried about was not malignant, she asked me if there was anything I could suggest to relieve her dry facial skin. I gave her a number of suggestions regarding moisturizers, soaps, water temperature for washing and rinsing, exfoliation, explaining what sorts of cosmetics she should use and which she should avoid. Another woman, whom I was treating for a persistent rash on her hands, mentioned in passing that her hair had begun to break off. I reviewed with her the procedures and products she could use to help her minimize the breakage and improve the condition of her hair. Patients come in about acne and then ask about stretch marks or wrinkles. Or they'll want to know if I think a particular new cosmetic would be right for them.

Many times, they'll describe a familiar problem that can turn into a "beauty crisis": puffy eyes on the morning of an important meeting. A cold sore just before a big date. Then they'll ask what to do if the problem recurs.

Despite the questions, a few patients seem surprised when I have the answers to problems that are purely cosmetic. When I gave one patient a "recipe" for an exfoliating treatment to brighten her skin, she said, "I just thought I'd mention how dull my skin looked; I wasn't sure you'd be able to help." The truth is we don't have courses in "treating" tired-looking skin in medical school. But a thorough grounding in the structure and functioning of skin, hair, and nails enables the dermatologist to offer effective solutions to everyday and not-so-common beauty problems. Though I don't do hair removal, for example, I know that because of variations in skin structure and sensitivity, some hair-removal products and techniques are a better choice for certain areas of the body than others. And because certain beauty problems are also medical problems— like the unsightly fungal infection that can be caused by artificial nails—the dermatologist can offer the safest and most effective beauty remedies.

My patients don't usually come in to see me about nonmedical beauty problems; nevertheless, they're eager for the safe, unbiased, scientifically sound solutions that only a dermatologist can provide. You won't find here any routine advice on daily upkeep of skin, hair, and nails. Instead I focus on how to deal with beauty problems. I tell you what to do in an emergency—when a sudden, mysterious rash or blemish prevents you from looking your best, for example—and I provide recommendations that make future emergencies less likely. I tell you how to self-treat a range of "chronic" conditions from skimpy hair (or too much hair where you don't want it) to weak nails to excessive perspiration to skin that's super dry or oily. I pass on a variety of special facials and other treatments you can give yourself at home to minimize signs of aging today and tell you what you can do now to ensure younger looks in the future.

Just as important, I tell you what not to do, because the wrong course of action will only compound the problem. And of course I help you determine when and if a problem is beyond self-treatment and needs medical attention from a dermatologist or other doctor.

Many of my patients have found themselves confused by the enormous variety of cosmetics that are available. Therefore, I include information on how to choose products appropriate to different skin types and conditions and guidelines on how to get the best results from those products. Equally important, I let you know which ingredients in products are potential troublemakers for *you* and how you can avoid them.

I answer some of the most-asked questions about those high-tech "anti-aging" creams, lotions, and gels you've been hearing so much about, and cue you in on what you can reasonably expect from them. I also explain the principles behind wrinkle fixers such as injectible collagen, Retin-A, Fibrel, silicone, and microlipectomy, and help you determine which, if any, are for you.

Why a beauty book by a doctor? So that you can have direct, instant access to dermatologically sound, speedy remedies and longer-term solutions exactly when you need it.

And because, for so many women, the sudden blossoming of a pimple is the most dreaded, common beauty emergency, what better place to start than with how to nip a blemish in the early stages?

THE DOCTOR'S BEAUTY HOTLINE

1

Fast Fixes for Pimples and Oily Skin

If you think twenty-one is the magic age at which pimples suddenly cease to be a problem, you are wrong.

Though acne is most prevalent among adolescents, many mature women in their thirties, forties, even fifties, are bothered by an occasional blemish. (In fact, adult acne seems to be on the rise. Dermatological studies indicate it's about 60 percent more common now than it was a decade ago.) If frantic calls for emergency help from my patients are any indication, pimples have a way of surfacing at exactly the wrong time. "Just when I have to look my best, my skin breaks out." I hear this all the time.

I use the term *pimple* rather loosely here to refer to a variety of blemishes: *papules*, the red, sometimes tender pimples that have not yet come to a head; *pustules*, mature, white-capped pimples; and cystlike pimples, those angry, inflamed eruptions that are more deeply rooted in the skin.

The simple self-treatments described in this chapter will help calm the occasional flare-up and speed its disappearance. The preventive measures I recommend should help control oily skin (which is prone to develop pimples and blackheads) and reduce the likelihood of future flare-ups. But if pimples are chronic, face up to the fact that your problem is *acne*, and that you need professional help from a dermatologist. I urge you to get it.

With that caveat in mind, here's how to self-treat a pimple or two.

Common Pimples (Papules)

The following procedure has helped many of my patients clear up the occasional round, reddish bump.

1. Wash your face with mild soap and lukewarm water. Rinse thoroughly with cool water and blot dry with a fresh towel.
2. Crack or crush several ice cubes; place them in a plastic sandwich bag or wrap in a clean washcloth.
3. Apply ice to the bump. Hold it in place for as long as you can stand the cold. (Try for ten minutes.)
4. Remove the ice and dot on an over-the-counter acne medication containing 5 percent benzoyl peroxide. Confine application to the pimple. These products are drying and can cause peeling or irritation in surrounding skin, especially if your skin tends to be sensitive.
5. Repeat every four hours or so until the bump has diminished in size and is no longer red.

Pre-makeup disguise for a pimple. It's better not to wear makeup over a pimple, but if you feel you must, first dot the blemish with a tinted acne medication such as Clinique's Anti-Acne Control formula or Noxzema's Clear-Up Acne Medicine. Allow it to dry, then apply makeup as usual.

TIP: If the area around the pimple is very red and tinted medication doesn't tone it down, mix a drop of liquid or cream concealer with a drop of foundation and blend it over the redness. Then proceed with makeup.

Keep in mind that *noncomedogenic cosmetics*—those free of oil and other common acne-instigating ingredients—are best if you are troubled with occasional blemishes.

Mature Pimples (Pustules)

The following treatment can help reduce inflammation and facilitate drainage of white-capped pimples that have come to a head:

1. Wash with mild soap and lukewarm water. Rinse thoroughly with warm water and blot dry with a clean towel.

2. Boil three or four pints of water and pour into a large bowl. Tent a towel over your head, bend close to the bowl, and steam your face for five minutes.

3. When the water has cooled slightly, add one tablespoon of salt per pint of water and stir to mix.

4. Test to make sure the water is cool enough not to burn, then saturate a cotton ball or gauze square in the mixture, press out excess, and apply to pimple for a minute or so. Repeat several times.

5. Saturate cotton ball or gauze in witch hazel or rubbing alcohol and apply to pimple with very gentle pressure for thirty seconds. Blot dry.

6. Repeat the entire procedure several times during the day and into the evening. If the pimple's white cap is dislodged during the steam/soak process, do not attempt to press out the contents. Continue to steam and soak until leakage or oozing has stopped and the pimple is dry. Once or twice more should do it.

Cover-up techniques for a pustule. If the white cap is off and the pimple is still moist, do not use makeup on it; to do so could result in infection. Instead, when it's time to get ready for work or a social engagement, dot the pimple with a tinted medicated cream or lotion, such as those listed for camouflaging papules. (Other good choices are Liquimat Lotion, which comes in a variety of shades, and Acnotex Lotion.) If you like, apply your usual makeup around, but not directly to, the pimple.

When you're back home again, resume the steam/soak treat-

ment until the pimple is dry. At that point, it's safe to use
foundation makeup over a tinted medicated product.

Cystlike Pimples

If you've ever had one, you know the warning signs: localized
soreness and perhaps a throbbing sensation or a feeling of
warmth in the area beginning hours or even a day or so before
redness and swelling are visible on the surface.

Cystlike pimples originate well below the surface of the skin,
in the layer called the *dermis*, which contains blood vessels,
oil, and sweat glands. The deep-rootedness of these lesions
helps explain why they sometimes take so long to erupt. When
they finally do, it's often with a vengeance. These typically
large, angry-looking, painful blemishes may linger for days or
weeks and sometimes leave scars to remember them by. (If a
membrane, or sac, forms around the contents and a true cyst
develops, it may never go away without dermatological intervention.)

You have two options. You can wait it out and allow the
pimple to run its course, while you hope for the best: quick
healing, no scarring. (A tinted medicated cream or lotion can
be applied to help conceal the problem.) Or you can see a
dermatologist. He or she may recommend treatment with a
dilute synthetic steroid derivative, such as Kenalog. The solution, injected directly into the lesion with a very fine-gauge
needle, often prevents cystlike pimples from "ripening" fully,
eases redness and soreness, and may shrink blemishes signifi-
cantly, often within a day or two.

What Not to Do About a Pimple

Following the above procedures and tips should prove helpful
to most people most of the time. At best, they provide almost

instant improvement. And at the very least, the appropriate treatment helps shorten the lifespan of a blemish.

Unfortunately, that's not the case with many other self-help treatments. Some do a lot more harm than good. In fact, in my opinion, the don'ts of treating a pimple are as important as the dos. Here are four crucial don'ts.

• Don't pick or squeeze. I can't emphasize this point enough. I *know* what a temptation it is to use your fingers or one of those drugstore devices to try to get rid of a pimple, especially after it has come to a head. Nevertheless, don't do it! It doesn't matter how clean your hands are, rough handling of any kind— even resting your face in the palms of your hands!—increases irritation in the area and can result in greater inflammation or infection and add to the risk of scarring.

• Don't use harsh, abrasive cleansing methods on skin break-outs. The occasional blemish isn't caused by surface dirt. And neither is a full-blown case of acne. Using a rough washcloth, brush, or polyester facial sponge to scrub and rub at a pimple can have much the same effect as picking and squeezing: skin in the area may become more sensitive and inflamed, and as a result, healing may take longer than if you'd left it alone. Not to mention the fact that overzealous cleansing can trigger an increase in oil producton, setting the stage for future blem-ishes.

There may be times when gentle abrasion can be used to "wake up" your skin and give it a healthy glow. But not now, when you are fighting a pimple.

• Don't try to hide blemishes under heavy foundation makeup or concealer. Many products that provide good coverage con-tain ingredients that can aggravate existing pimples and/or in-vite the development of new ones. Do not use foundation of any kind over an "open," moist blemish.

• Don't make the mistake of assuming that your skin is oily— and treating it that way—just because you get a pimple now and then. As I'll explain in the next section, oil *is* a factor in the development of a blemish, and oily skin *is* more prone to

breakouts than other skin types, but it is not uncommon for
people with normal or even dry skin to experience a flare-up
from time to time.

Unfortunately, I've seen patients with normal and dry skin
who dealt with an occasional pimple by using aggressive tactics
intended for oily-skin care. The scrubs and astringents and the
potent degreasers really did a job on their skin; their faces
looked raw and dehydrated. And the pimples they thought they
were fighting were still there!

If your skin is indeed oily, you'll benefit from products formulated for oily skin and the oily-skin care tips you'll find later
in this chapter. But if it's normal or dry, oily-skin cleansers and
other products can strip it of the moisture it needs to stay fresh
and young looking.

Use products keyed to your skin type, whatever it is.

Blackheads

Though nowhere near as traumatic as a pimple, a scattering of
blackheads is not flattering. Usually, I tell patients who are
bothered by blackheads to try gentle exfoliation with a product
keyed to their skin type. Almost every major beauty company
markets these products. Product names tend to include the
words "exfoliating," "sloughing," or "clarifying," and commonly used ingredients are salicylic acid, resorcinol, sulphur,
or benzoyl peroxide. The products work by dissolving the top
layer of old dead skin cells, after which blackheads may be
loosened enough to be washed away. An exfoliating mask (many
of these are made of clay) has the same effect.

When you want to get rid of a single troublesome blackhead,
resist the temptation to squeeze it out. I've already explained
why squeezing is harmful. Don't do it. There's a better way:

1. Wash your face with mild soap and warm water. Rinse
and pat dry.

2. Pour boiling water into a large bowl or the bathroom basin. Tent a towel over your head, and, keeping your face at least twelve inches from the water, steam for five to ten minutes.

3. Dip a sterile gauze pad into the water (it should still be very warm, but not hot enough to burn), press out excess moisture, and hold it against the blackhead for another two minutes.

4. With a fresh gauze pad wrapped around each index finger, exert gentle pressure on the skin on either side of the blackhead. Most blackheads will pop out after such pressure is applied. *Do not force the issue by squeezing or picking.*

5. Splash the area with cold water. Then dab with a cotton ball soaked in witch hazel or rubbing alcohol.

6. Wait at least an hour, or until all redness and swelling have disappeared, before applying makeup.

7. If you were unsuccessful in getting rid of the blackhead, you might try "priming" it with a dot of a benzoyl peroxide product applied several times a day for a few days. Then try again, as above.

IMPORTANT: Do not attempt to remove more than one blackhead per session. Allow a few days to pass before going after a second one.

Whiteheads

Never use physical means of any kind to attempt to dislodge a whitehead. The possibility of scarring is just too great. To treat a whitehead, dot on an over-the-counter acne medication containing benzoyl peroxide. With repeated use over time, benzoyl peroxide may peel and dissolve the thin layer of skin that covers the pore, allowing the contents—sebum— to escape. Of course, if whiteheads are numerous and acne medication fails to clear them up, you should see your dermatologist.

Biography of a Blemish

"Why me? Why now?" I hear these words time and again from frustrated patients who have to deal with sudden, unexpected skin flare-ups. You've probably said it yourself.

To understand the whys of a blemish, you need to know how it gets its start. To simplify, one or more of a wide range of factors—hormonal, environmental, or both—stimulate oil glands within the skin to produce more oil. At the same time, cells lining the pores may become thicker and more numerous, in effect narrowing pore openings. When oil, dead skin cells, and bacteria are trapped within a pore, the result can be what doctors call a *microcomedo*, which may become enlarged and develop into a *closed comedo* (a whitehead) or an *open comedo* (blackhead). If the buildup of white blood cells martialed to combat the bacteria in the pore is great enough to rupture the walls of the pore, the result can be further inflammation and a pimple (papule or pustule), which sometimes develops into a larger lesion called a *nodule* or *cyst*.

Whiteheads and blackheads are solid plugs composed of oil and cell debris lodged in pore openings. A whitehead is "closed"; skin has grown over the opening of the pore, making it impossible for the contents to move out. A blackhead is "open" and lodges at the surface of the skin. (The dark color of a blackhead has little to do with dirt; rather, it is caused by melanin, the substance that gives skin its color, and by oxidation, which occurs when the oily plug is exposed to air.)

A papule begins when trapped oil, debris, bacteria, and white blood cells (pus) burst through follicle walls into the surrounding dermis.

A pustule is a papule that has come to a head.

A cyst is the result of a large amount of debris rupturing follicle walls deep within the dermis.

Now let's take a closer look at some of the factors and circumstances that can trigger the development of a blemish.

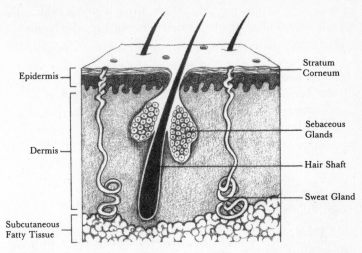

Simplified cross section of the skin shows the stratum corneum, composed of dead skin cells, the epidermis, and the dermis. The dermis contains sweat glands, hair follicles, and attached sebaceous glands.

The Instigators

It's sometimes easier to track down the cause of a moderate to severe case of acne than to pinpoint the instigator(s) of an occasional pimple. Still, the more you know about the products, habits, circumstances, and environmental influences with blemish-producing potential, the better your chances of figuring out which ones might be contributing to your problems. Then you can make changes that will benefit your skin.

Cosmetics and toiletries. Many women wear too much, and too many different kinds of products, on their faces. Not all cosmetics are villains. However, a wide range are made with substances that are known to be *comedogenic*—that is, they can block pores or affect the cells lining the skin's oil glands in ways that promote the development of pimples. Some potential troublemakers are listed below. If you've been using a product containing one or more of them, see what happens when you switch to a similar product made without ingredients on the suspect list.

acetol acetulan   crude coal tar
acetylated lanolin   D & C red dyes (often
amberate P   found in blusher)
butyl stearate   decyl oleate

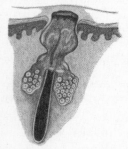

A blackhead forms when a follicle becomes clogged with cell debris and a backup of sebum that enlarges the pore opening. The dark color is due to the presence of melanin, the substance that gives skin its color.

A papule results when an accumulation of cell debris and sebum narrows a pore opening, becomes trapped within a follicle, and breaks through the follicle's "walls." A papule appears as a reddish bump on the surface of the skin.

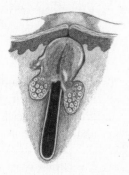

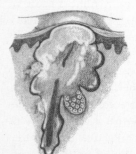

When white blood cells invade the material within a follicle, pus is formed and the result is a pustule (a pimple that has "come to a head").

ethyloxylated lanolin
isocetyl stearate
isopropyl isostearate
isopropyl lanolate
isopropyl myristate
isopropyl palmitate
isostearyl neopentanoate

langogene
lanosterin
myristyl myristate
octyl palmitate
octyl stearate
PG 2 myristyl propionate
sterolan

In addition to the substances above, the following cosmetic and toiletry ingredients can cause problems when used frequently, over a period of time. Avoid them if possible:

hexadecyl alcohol
hexylene glycol
lanolins
polyethylene glycol
sodium laurel sulfate

One way to keep most or all of these troublemakers from coming into contact with your skin is to use products labeled "noncomedogenic." Many companies specialize in noncomedogenic makeup and skin-care preparations; others include noncomedogenic alternatives to the products in their regular lines. To help prevent those once-in-a-while blemishes, you might want to consider the following cosmetics.

FOUNDATIONS

Adrien Arpel Glycerine Liquid Powder
Allercreme Oil-Free
Almay Fresh Look Oil-Free Makeup
Almay Oil-Control Makeup for Oily Skin
Clinique Pore Minimizer
Elizabeth Arden Extra Control for Problem Skin
Estée Lauder Demi-Matte Makeup Oil-Free
Estée Lauder Fresh Air Makeup Base
Lancôme Maquicontrôle Oil-Free Liquid Makeup

Maybelline Shine Free Oil Control Makeup
Prescriptives Exact Color Makeup 100% Oil-Free

BLUSHER

Almay Brush-On Blush
Clinique Young Face Powder Blush
Max Factor Maxi-Unshine 100% Oil Free Blushing Powder
Maybelline Shine Free Powder Blush

FACE POWDERS

Almay Translucent Pressed Powder
Corn Silk Loose Powder
Corn Silk Pressed Powder
Estée Lauder Demi-Matte Loose Powder Oil-Free
Estée Lauder Demi-Matte Pressed Powder Oil-Free
Maybelline Shine Free Oil Control Dual Powder Base

MOISTURIZERS

Allercreme
Almay
Aquaderm Cream
Complex 15
Keri Facial Cleanser
Moisturel
Neutrogena
Nutraderm
Prescriptives Oil-Free Skin Renewer Lotion

Pressure. Leaning your chin into your hands, absentmindedly stroking or rubbing your cheeks or even wearing a sweatband, can ignite flare-ups.

The theory goes something like this: Pressure prevents moisture from evaporating from the skin's surface, causing cells to become "waterlogged" and to swell. As a result, pore openings are reduced in size, and oil, instead of flowing out to the surface where it can be washed away, becomes trapped. It's this trapped oil that makes blemishes more likely.

If pimples always seem to occur in the same area, stop and think. Do you, consciously or unconsciously, apply pressure to that area? Lean on it? Rub it? If the answer is yes, try to break the habit.

An "oily" environment. Men and women who are exposed to large amounts of oil or grease on the job or in their leisure hours do not always realize that the oil acts as a kind of catalyst for blemishes.

If you work in or near the cooking area of a restaurant (especially the fast-food kind, with burgers always sizzling on the grill), or use machine oil or other types of grease on the job or in your spare time, it's a good bet that your environment is a contributing factor to skin breakouts. Wash frequently, wear only noncomedogenic cosmetics—and if breakouts are chronic, see a dermatologist for treatment and preventive measures.

Food and vitamins. A diet high in iodide- and/or flouride-rich foods tends to promote blemishes. Among the foods to watch out for are shellfish and spinach, beef liver, asparagus, and, of course, iodized salt. (Kelp and seaweed, though not commonly eaten in this country, are also notorious pimple instigators.) Incidentally, you might be surprised to learn, as many of my patients are, that chocolate does not appear to aggravate acne.

Vitamin B_{12} injections, sometimes used to treat anemia, can also cause flare-ups. (B_{12} preparations may contain small amounts of iodine.) If you are being given such injections, discuss the matter with your doctor.

Medications. A variety of prescription and over-the-counter drugs are formulated with substances that promote pimples. A short list of such drugs follows:

> aspirin and products made with salicylates (such as Alka-Seltzer, Fiorinal, ibuprofin, Midol, Pepto-Bismol)
> asthma and cold remedies containing bromides or iodides

corticosteroids taken orally (and, occasionally, high-potency
   topically applied corticosteroids)
low-estrogen birth control pills containing progesterone

Of course, serious medical considerations must take prece-
dence over minor skin problems, and you may have to continue a course of treatment that causes occasional skin
blemishes. However, why not talk it over with your doctor? He
or she may be able to prescribe alternative drugs formulated
without the skin-offending ingredients.

Heat, humidity, sun. Soaring temperatures and moisture-laden
air boost sweat and oil production, and the result can be one,
two, or a whole crop of pimples. You can counteract these
environmental influences with frequent, gentle cleansing.

If lathering up with soap and water at midday is inconven-
ient, at least remove grime and stale makeup with an antiseptic
lotion, such as Noxzema's Antiseptic Skin Cleanser.

Sun exposure, without excessive sweating, tends to dry surface oils and promote skin peeling, both of which tend to be
pimple inhibiting. Nevertheless, my office is often jam-packed
with acne patients in early autumn, just as the sunbathing season ends. I suspect that the buildup of dead skin cells as a result
of prolonged sunbathing clogs pores and follicles; pimples are
the eventual consequence. One way to prevent this scenario is
to use a noncomedogenic sunscreen at the beach. (In Chapter
9, I discuss why daily sunscreening, throughout the year, is important.)

Stress. Tension, frustration, impatience, anxiety—all can show
up on skin in the form of blemishes. How does this happen?
In many cases, stress alters the balance of hormones in the
body. Estrogen levels may decrease while progesterone and
other hormones stay the same or increase. These changes can
stimulate oil glands to produce more oil. When that happens,
the stage is set for a breakout.

If stress seems to be getting the better of you and your skin, you're not alone. I'm seeing more and more women, many of them just entering or reentering the workforce, or recently promoted to more responsible, high-powered jobs, whose skin problems seem to be related to this.

My advice to them and to you is to learn how to manage stress. Exercise, for example, is a great way to let off steam, calm your nerves, ease your mind. (Next time you feel the tension level escalating, why not get out for a brisk ten-minute walk?) For more information about stress management, pick up one of the many excellent books on the subject. Or visit a stress clinic. There's one in almost every community now. Most large hospitals and university medical schools operate stress clinics, as do many Ys and health clubs.

I've emphasized various pimple-promoting factors here for the same reason I do it in the office, with my patients: To make you aware that skin breakouts aren't necessarily beyond your control, that they could be a consequence of something you're doing or not doing—and that altering your behavior and your environment might make a big difference.

A case in point: A model in her late twenties—I'll call her Joanna—came to see me about a recurring crop of "mysterious" pimples that appeared only on her forehead. (The rest of her skin was smooth and very clear.) She had been to another dermatologist, who recommended treating the area with a benzoyl peroxide product. It was good advice; the breakouts were less severe now. But even a few small blemishes were enough to interfere with Joanna's livelihood. She wanted better results.

When I see pimples on the forehead, I immediately check out the patient's hairstyle: bangs, or hair worn swept across the brow can cause problems. Hair didn't seem to be a factor in this case, since Joanna wore hers off her face. We sat down and I took her through the list of common troublemakers, one by one. None of them seemed to apply. However, as we talked, she leaned back in her chair and began to massage her fore-head.

"Do you do that often?" I asked. "Do what?" she said. She was completely unaware that she was rubbing her forehead. But when I pointed it out to her, she realized it was something she did often when she was trying to concentrate or feeling tired. On a hunch, I asked her if she used hand cream. It turned out that she did—and that it was one containing lanolin, which is a comedogen.

I gave her the names of several hand creams that are less comedogenic and suggested that she make an effort to stop massaging her forehead. The "mysterious" pimples are a thing of the past.

For Joanna, the problem was almost certainly the lanolin in her hand cream that she was unconsciously rubbing into her forehead. For you, it might be one or a combination of a num-ber of other factors. Be sure to give the factors listed earlier in this section serious consideration.

Your genetic makeup. Of course, there are some things that can't be changed. Certain people are simply more likely than others to have troubled skin. It's in their genes. Since there's nothing you can do about your genetic makeup, you should be espe-cially wary of products, habits, and environmental factors that contribute to breakouts and avoid as many as you can. If and when blemishes get out of hand, by all means see a dermatol-ogist. Almost all acne can be controlled now. For the ways and means, take a look at my book, *Your Skin: A Dermatologist's Guide to a Lifetime of Beauty and Health.*

Special Care Tips for Blemished Skin

The quick self-help measures for pimples suggested earlier are fine as emergency treatments. Even more important in con-trolling and preventing blemishes is the routine care you give your skin. Here's what I recommend to patients with a tendency to break out:

• Wash your face morning and evening, and if convenient, at midday too, with lukewarm water and mild soap or cleansing bar, such as Purpose, Lowila Cake, Aveenobar, or Dove. Use your fingertips only. Do not scrub with a washcloth, brush, or sponge. If flare-ups are frequent, you might want to try a medicated soap (these are often labeled "antimicrobial" or "bacteriostatic") or one containing sulfur. If your skin is dry, use it on pimple-prone areas only. Rinse thoroughly by splashing ten to twelve times with lukewarm water. Blot dry by patting gently with a clean towel.

• Don't use moisturizer on blemishes. Instead, apply an astringent with a sterile cotton ball. Witch hazel is a good choice. Avoid astringents and skin fresheners that are pore minimizers. In plumping up surrounding skin cells, they constrict pore openings and can interfere with the free flow of oil to the surface, thus adding to your problems.

• Important enough to repeat: Use only noncomedogenic cosmetics. Labels will help you determine which belong in this category.

• Consider treating the areas where breakouts are most likely to occur (this could mean your entire face) with a tinted drying cream or lotion containing sulfur, resorcinol, and/or salicylic acid. A few examples follow:

Acnederm Lotion
Acnomel Cream
Clearasil Adult Acne Care Medicated Blemish Cream
Pernox Lotion
Rezamid
Liquimat Lotion
Night Cast—R
Night Cast—S

These products work to dry and peel away upper layers of skin cells and are often remarkably effective in getting rid of existing pimples. Use according to instructions on the label, being careful not to allow the product to come into contact with delicate skin around the eyes, under the chin, and on the neck.

IMPORTANT: If your skin is black or dark, do not use formulas containing sulfur and resorcinol unless prescribed by a dermatologist, because these ingredients can cause changes in skin pigmentation.

• You might want to try products containing benzoyl peroxide as the active ingredient. These penetrate pores to kill bacteria that cause pimples and also act as peeling agents; they accelerate healing of blemishes and help prevent new ones if applied regularly to areas where they tend to crop up. Among the best benzoyl peroxide medications are Topex Gel, Oxy 5 and Oxy 10, and Clearasil benzoyl peroxide formulations.

Before you buy, check the percentage of benzoyl peroxide in a product. The range in over-the-counter formulas is from 2.5 to 10 percent. If your skin is dry or sensitive, or if you are very fair, start with the 2.5 formulation. Otherwise, begin with a product containing 5 percent benzoyl peroxide. In any case, choose a water-based lotion or gel-type formulation rather than one with an oil base. (Some of the latter contain comedogenic ingredients that can promote new pimples!) Don't forget to check the expiration date stamped on the package; these products have a fairly short shelf life.

You may have to build up tolerance to benzoyl peroxide, especially if your skin is sensitive. Apply a small amount at first and wash it off after three hours. (If applied lightly, it can be worn under makeup.) Gradually work up to using more of the product for longer periods. *Some* irritation and dryness are unavoidable and in fact indicate that the benzoyl peroxide is doing what it's supposed to do. But a harsh stinging or burning sensation and extreme peeling are signals to stop using it for a day or two. When you resume, cut back on the amount and the time you wear it. (Conversely, if there is no peeling and not even a slight tingling, try applying more of the product and wearing it for longer periods or consider switching to a product with a higher percentage of benzoyl peroxide.)

For best results, wait at least thirty minutes after washing before using benzoyl peroxide. Avoid sensitive areas around the eyes, on the neck, near the nostrils, earlobes, lips, and corners of the mouth. Since the peeling action leaves skin especially vulnerable to sun damage, don't go out without a sunscreen or makeup containing sunscreening ingredients. Most important, unless you experience uncomfortable rawness and inflammation, keep at it. It takes about a month before improvement is noticeable.

• Wash your hair frequently—at least every other day and preferably daily. Use a gentle shampoo keyed to your hair type. Avoid using heavy, creamy, or oily conditioners and styling products, even if your hair is dry (whether naturally or because of abuse). These can aggravate pimple problems especially in the forehead area. (In fact, heavy hair dressings are sometimes a *cause* of forehead blemishes.)

Best hairstyles are those that clear your face. If you've been wearing bangs, sweep them to the side or keep them off your face with a headband.

• Don't wear cosmetics to exercise class or during tennis or other sports since excessive perspiration plus makeup is a recipe for pimples if you are blemish-prone. (Do, however, wear an oil-free sunscreen for out-of-door workouts.) Wash your face and shower with a gentle soap after physical activity. Launder sweatbands, leotards, tennis whites, and other exercise clothing after every wearing. The combination of oil, perspiration, and grime that accumulates on them can irritate and aggravate existing skin problems and bring on new ones. (It's a good idea to have at least two of everything so you'll always have fresh exercise gear to slip into.)

When to See a Dermatologist

There's a lot you can do on your own to combat the occasional pimple and to make blemishes less likely to occur in the future. However, if skin flare-ups are frequent or becoming more so, if your skin is tender or inflamed, if your pimples sometimes leave scars, you need more help.

I suffered with acne when I was younger, and my daughters are acne-prone today, so the treatment of this disorder has always been a special interest of mine. I'm happy to say that we dermatologists have an increasingly sophisticated and effective arsenal of acne fighters at our disposal. Though no doctor can promise you'll have the complexion of your dreams within a few months of your first appointment (we deal in medicine, not magic), there are few cases that don't respond to a customized approach, which might include a combination of treatments. Your doctor, for example, might fight acne with oral antibiotics, topically applied antibiotics, vitamin A acid, benzoyl peroxide, corticosteroid injections, hormone therapy, liquid nitrogen, dry ice (used to peel away upper layers of skin), ultraviolet light, acne surgery (for blackheads), peeling solutions or pastes, and in severe cases of disfiguring cystic acne, Accutane. Help is available. It's there when you need it.

Quick Help for Oily Skin

There's at least one advantage to having oily skin: because it has its own plentiful supply of natural moisturizers in the form of *sebum* (oil), it tends to wrinkle less and at a later age than other skin types. (Skin oils do not, however, have a delaying effect on other signs of aging, such as sagging and loss of tone).

As for the disadvantages, you're no doubt already well aware of them. Excess oil shows up as an unattractive, greasy shine that makes skin look less than fresh and clean. If oil flow is really heavy, it can "soak" through makeup, causing it to wear off quickly and even change color. And of course when oil combines with the debris of dead skin cells, it can contribute to blocked pores, leading to pimples and blackheads.

There's no safe and easy way to control oil production from within (through diet, for example), but you can remove the excess from without and minimize the greasy appearance.

Oil Blotters

Clay masks absorb oil and help tone down shine, leaving skin looking fresher and cleaner. When selecting a commercial mask, keep in mind that as a general rule, the darker the clay, the more absorbent it will be. Dark brown and green clays are best for oily skin. There are also some good gel-type (peel-off) masks that help loosen blackheads and clear away excess oil. Be sure to read labels to find out which masks are recommended for oily skin.

Or you might want to try concocting your own anti-oil facials. Here are two do-it-yourself masks to try:

Thirty-Five-Minute Mask to Blot Up Excess Oil

You'll need some yeast for this one—either a cake of brewer's yeast or a packet of active dry yeast.

1. Wash your face, rinse with warm water, and pat dry.
2. In a small bowl, mix yeast with enough water to form a spreadable paste.
3. With your fingers, scoop up the yeast mixture and smooth evenly onto your face, avoiding eyelids, the undereye area, and your mouth. Leave on for about half an hour.
4. Rinse with warm water. When all traces of yeast are gone, splash eight to ten times with very cool water.
5. Finish with an astringent or skin toner made for oily skin or with a greaseless moisturizer if you use one.

Eight-Minute Facial to Take Off the Slick

The main ingredient in this oil-control treatment is milk of magnesia. Any brand will do.

1. Wash your face, rinse with warm water, and pat dry.
2. Pour two tablespoons of milk of magnesia into a bowl. Dab onto face with a cotton ball or gauze pad, avoiding eye and mouth areas. Wait five to six minutes.

3. Remove milk of magnesia by rinsing your face with warm water. Then splash several more times with very cool water.

4. Apply astringent, toner, or greaseless moisturizer.

TIP: For even better oil control, cleanse your face, then *steam*, before applying a mask.

Exfoliation

Oily skin tends to be thick. And because it's thick, it may appear to be more sallow, or "pasty," than other skin types, since the pinkness of the blood-rich dermis below the surface does not show through.

Regular, frequent removal of upper layers of dead skin cells—exfoliation—will not thin your skin enough to make a real, permanent difference. But it will help prevent excessive dead-cell buildup—a factor in pimple production—and bring blood nearer to the surface so that your complexion takes on a rosier color, at least temporarily.

If your skin is oily but blemish free, you can exfoliate by physical means with—in ascending order of harshness—a soft washcloth, a complexion brush, or a polyester facial sponge. But don't just scrub away at your skin. Dampen your face, lather up with soap or a detergent bar, then gently massage suds onto skin with the exfoliator, moving it in smallish circles. Do not apply enough pressure to pull or drag at your skin. Don't massage for prolonged periods (a minute should be enough). And do not exfoliate at all if your skin is broken out. You can exfoliate as above as often as your skin can take it. If soreness, excessive redness, or irritation develops, cut back or stop completely for a few days.

Two-Minute Salt-and-Soap Exfoliation

For more aggressive, once- or twice-a-week exfoliation, you might want to try the following. You'll need two teaspoons of ordinary table salt and your regular soap or detergent bar.

1. If you are wearing makeup, remove it with a cotton ball or gauze pad moistened with a light oil or commercial makeup remover.

2. Wet your face by splashing with warm water.

3. With your hands, work soap or detergent into a rich lather. Add half the salt and rub palms together.

4. *Glide* lather and salt onto your face with light, sweeping strokes, then gently massage forehead, cheeks, and chin. Work in smallish circles, using the balls of your fingertips only. Continue, adding more salt as necessary, for one minute.

5. Rinse thoroughly with warm water, gradually adjusting temperature to cold.

6. Pat dry with a soft towel. If you ordinarily apply an astringent or toner after washing, you can do so now. However, dab on just a little to start; if it stings, rinse it off and use a greaseless moisturizer instead. Later on, when your skin becomes accustomed to salt-and-soap exfoliation, you may be able to tolerate your usual follow-up astringent or toner.

Special Care Tips for Oily Skin

Cleansing

Obviously, when oil is too much of a good thing, frequent, proper cleansing is important. Wash your face twice a day, once in the morning and once at bedtime. "Touch-up" cleansing— either with soap and water or with cotton balls saturated in an astringent lotion—is advisable when the weather is hot and humid or if you work in a greasy environment (such as the kitchen of a fast-food restaurant). You should also remove excess oil with soap and water or an astringent after exercise or other activity that causes you to work up a sweat and before reapplying makeup for an afternoon or evening engagement.

If your complexion is extremely oily and occasional breakouts are a problem, consider using a soap containing sulfur, which helps dry up oil. Pernox is a good example. Soaps made with glycerine and alcohol also tend to be excellent choices for oily skin. Neutrogena's Oily Skin Formula Transparent Facial Bar is one. However, almost any good soap that is not super-fatted will do the job. (If ingredients such as cold cream, cocoa butter, coconut oil, and lanolin are mentioned on the label, the soap is superfatted.)

I don't believe in making a big production out of face wash-ing. At the same time, there's more to doing a good job on oily skin than just a quick lather and rinse.

1. If you are wearing makeup, remove it with a cotton ball and baby oil or with a commercial makeup remover.

2. Pre-wet your skin by splashing with very warm water.

3. Work soap into a lather and apply with your fingertips. If your skin is unblemished, you could use instead a soft wash-cloth, complexion brush, or facial sponge. Work in smallish circles. Don't neglect the areas around the hairline, under your jaw and neck.

4. Rinse thoroughly. Start by splashing with very warm wa-ter. Gradually adjust temperature to cool. Use only fresh run-ning water; don't fill the basin and splash repeatedly with the same water.

5. Blot dry with a clean, soft towel.

6. Apply an astringent, toner, or skin freshener formulated for oily skin, or use witch hazel. (Store these products in the refrigerator so they'll be well chilled when you use them.)

Oily *mature* skin often benefits from a light, oil-free moistur-izer, such as Neutrogena Moisture, at least on the delicate areas under eyes and around the mouth. Some light, greaseless prod-ucts contain ingredients that duplicate the skin's own moisture. Among these are Aquacare Lotion and U-Lactin.

Makeup and Treatment Products

Avoid using products that contain the following ingredients: mineral oil (except to remove makeup before cleansing), lan-olin, petrolatum, isopropyl myristate, stearates. These all promote greasiness and increase the likelihood of blackheads and breakouts.

The following ingredients, however, tend to be anti-oil: alcohol, allantoin, calamine, kaolin, titanium oxide, zinc oxide. Products made with them are usually good—or at least not bad—for oily skin.

Avoid wearing makeup with the word "moisturizing" in its name or prominently featured on the label. These formulations are made with oily ingredients that add shine to your skin and, if you are blemish-prone, contribute to pimples.

The best foundations for you are those with a water base. (If it separates in the bottle and you need to shake it before applying, it's water-based.) Clinique's Pore Minimizer Makeup, which is also fragrance-free, is one. Many companies market entire lines of makeup for oily skin; some of the foundations are not strictly speaking water-based, but they're certainly a better choice than the moisturizing formulations.

Use loose powder to set makeup and minimize shine. A clean puff is important if you have a tendency to break out. (You can "launder" fabric puffs in sudsy water. You can also buy puffs by the pack.)

Fight greasy makeup breakthrough during the day by blotting your face with special oil-absorbent tissues, sold in pharmacies, variety and department stores. In a pinch, you can use eyeglass wipes for this purpose. Follow with loose or pressed powder.

2

Rx *for* Dry Skin

A woman I've known for several years (she used to bring in her daughter for treatment for acne) came in to my office one day extremely upset about what she took to be sudden signs of aging. "Look at all these little wrinkles," she said, pointing to her cheeks and the areas around her eyes. "Overnight, I've got old-lady skin!"

She *did* look older than the last time I'd seen her, just a few weeks before. But the new lines and wrinkles on her face were not "overnight aging," as she believed. It was clear to me that somehow her usually normal-to-oily skin had undergone rapid and pronounced dehydration.

Sure enough, she'd just come back from a ski trip. Whole days spent out on the slopes, followed by evenings of sitting too close to a roaring fire, had stripped her skin of the moisture it needs to stay plumped up and "cushiony." Small but visible lines were the result.

Good, routine care over time can make a big difference to skin suddenly dried out through unusual circumstances, such as exposure to temperature extremes (indoor and outdoor) and dry environments—as in my patient's case—as well as to skin that is "naturally" dry. There are also some excellent, short-cut solutions that offer immediate, though temporary, results. Here are two of them.

Twenty-Minute Honey-Egg Moisturizing Mask

You'll need an egg yolk (rich in fatty cholesterol), some honey (a natural *humectant*, that is, a substance that attracts and holds moisture), and a moisturizing cream.

1. Remove makeup if you are wearing it. Use a cotton ball or gauze square and a light oil, such as baby oil.
2. Place the yolk of an egg and a tablespoon of honey in a cup and stir to mix.
3. Smooth egg-and-honey mixture onto your face, distributing it evenly on cheeks, forehead, nose, and chin. Do not apply to areas around eyes and mouth.
4. Wait fifteen minutes, then rinse thoroughly with tepid water.
5. Blot up excess moisture with a clean, soft towel. While skin is still slightly damp, apply a generous amount of moisturizer.

Ten-Minute Flake Fighter

Dryness often results in unattractive flaking of the skin. When that happens, this do-it-yourself facial can help smooth rough, flaky patches. Ingredients are baby oil, baking soda, and a moisturizer.

1. Remove makeup with a cotton ball or gauze square and a light oil, such as baby oil.
2. Pour about one-half teaspoon baby oil into the palm of one hand. Add enough baking soda to make a very thin paste. (Stir with your index finger.)
3. Apply to your face, "gliding" the mixture onto cheeks, forehead, nose, chin. Avoid eyelids and mouth. Work in small circles, using the lightest touch possible and spending no more than about ten seconds on any one area.
4. Rinse thoroughly with tepid water. Blot up excess water with a clean, soft towel. While skin is still slightly damp, apply a generous amount of moisturizing cream.

If your skin is very sensitive and feels sore or uncomfortable afterward, this procedure is obviously not for you. Do not repeat. However, if you like the results, you can deflake and moisturize, as above, once or twice a week.

Flakes and "False" Dryness

Once in a while someone with normal or oily skin will come to see me about persistent flakiness on the face, neck, or shoulders. The patient, assuming the problem is due to dryness, treats the flaking areas with a moisturizing cream or lotion— and instead of getting better, the condition worsens. By the time I see her (or him), we're looking at a full-blown case of *seborrheic dermatitis*, a nasty form of dandruff that can affect upper-body skin as well as the scalp. (For more information on seborrheic dermatitis, see Chapter 5.)

Don't automatically assume flakiness is a result of dryness. It might be. But if it doesn't respond to proper moisturizing (more about that in the next section) or seems to get worse, and certainly, if your skin shows no other signs of "dryness," see a dermatologist. Those flaking patches might be seborrheic dermatitis.

Everything You Always Wanted to Know About Moisturizers

They used to be known simply as "face creams" or sometimes "night creams." Then, a couple of decades ago, the word "moisturizers" came into vogue, and that's what these oil-in-water or water-in-oil products have been called ever since. "Moisturizers" is probably a better term for these creams and lotions since they are meant to smooth, soften, and plump up skin cells by means of hydration. They're your most important allies in combating dry skin.

A moisturizer works by retarding evaporation of water from the *stratum corneum*—upper layers of skin cells. These topmost cell layers must be composed of at least 10 percent water by volume to stay flexible and soft. When, through evaporation and lack of adequate replenishment of moisture from within, water content goes below 10 percent, skin becomes dry, flaky, dull looking, and rougher to the touch. Fine lines may become more noticeable.

Where does that all-important water in the stratum corneum come from? Most of the skin's natural moisture wells up from living cells deeper within the dermis. Externally applied water will moisturize temporarily, but as it evaporates, it can take some of the natural moisture already present in the skin along with it and result in greater dryness.

Oil is an important ingredient in moisturizing products not because it supplies moisture—water—but because, as you've often heard, oil and water don't mix. In fact, where water is concerned, oil is *occlusive*, meaning that it acts as a barrier. A coating of oil on the skin helps retard the evaporation of natural moisture from the stratum corneum. It also holds externally applied moisture in place against the skin.

In theory, just about any oily substance could be used as a moisturizer, including lard, shortening, cooking oil, unrefined lanolin, and petroleum jelly straight from the jar. However, they're aesthetically unacceptable, either because they're too heavy or because they have an unpleasant smell. Commercial moisturizers concocted by cosmetic chemists are formulated to be lighter, less greasy, and, except for those hypoallergenic products made without fragrance, pleasantly scented.

What's in Them?

Except for special-purpose products, the basic ingredients in facial moisturizers are all pretty much the same: oil and water. Light moisturizing products tend to be oil-in-water emulsions. Heavier moisturizing creams have more oil in them; as a result they're more occlusive and remain on the skin longer than lighter formulations. Many women like a lighter oil-in-water lotion for use under makeup and a heavier water-in-oil product for overnight moisturizing.

Some of the more common oils used in moisturizers are lanolin, mineral oil, petrolatum, cocoa butter, isopropyl myristate, and dimethicone.

Humectants, which attract water and hold it in contact with the skin, are important ingredients in many moisturizers. Glycerin, urea, lactic acid, and propylene glycol are all humectants.

Other no-frills ingredients include emulsifiers, which help prevent oily and nonoily ingredients from separating; thickeners, used to achieve and maintain desired consistency; preservatives and stabilizers to keep products fresh and discourage chemical breakdown due to microorganisms; and dyes and fragrances to enhance eye and nose appeal.

A number of additional ingredients are included in some moisturizing formulas. Many are featured on labels to attract the interest and attention of you, the consumer. However, in talking to my patients, I find there's a great deal of confusion about some of these substances—what they are, what they're good for, and why. You may have wondered about some of these ingredients too. Here's a brief rundown:

Aloe or aloe vera. This is a plant extract with slight soothing and healing properties.

Collagen. Almost 85 percent of skin is composed of interlaced collagen, a fibrous protein. Collagen is responsible for the wonderful firmness and tone of young skin. With age, as the underlying collagen begins to deteriorate, skin loses support from below. The top layers then begin to "collapse," and the result is loss of firmness and eventually sagging and heavy wrinkling. Collagen used as an ingredient in moisturizers is derived from cattle but is very similar to human collagen. However, the collagen in these products does not penetrate the skin and cannot augment your own natural supply. That's not to say that topically applied collagen has no value; it can add to the effectiveness of a moisturizer by binding water to the stratum corneum. (*Injectible* collagen is something else again. It can and does "erase" fine wrinkles and certain types of acne scars. For more about it, see Chapter 9.)

Elastin. Another fibrous component of the dermis, elastin is interwoven with collagen fibers to form a tight-knit, springy substratum for the skin. Like collagen, with the passage of years, elastin gradually deteriorates and skin becomes less resilient. As an ingredient in moisturizers and other treatment products, elastin does not penetrate and has no beneficial effect on skin tone and elasticity. But it is good at holding moisture within the upper layers of skin cells.

Jojoba. A plant extract commonly used in moisturizing products because of its ability to help heal, soothe, and soften.

NMF. Not a single ingredient but a mix, which together are identified by the term "natural moisturizing factor," because they are similar in chemical makeup to the moisture in human skin. Current dermatological opinion is that NMF is primarily a marketing gimmick.

Urea. Though it is an ingredient in many moisturizers, I haven't noticed it prominently featured on labels. I've included it here because it is a particularly valuable substance that promotes shedding of dead skin cells and encourages water absorption and retention. Some pharmacies sell inexpensive urea-based moisturizing products in foil packets.

Vitamins A, D, and E. As you might expect, topically applied vitamins do not "nourish" the skin. Their presence in moisturizing products is due mainly to their *oiliness*. Because of the effectiveness of Retin-A, made with vitamin A acid, in reversing some types of sun-related skin damage (including wrinkling), we're seeing vitamin A featured more and more prominently as an ingredient in cosmetics and treatment products. However, vitamin A, by itself, is not a skin rejuvenator. The wonder worker is tretinoin, the vitamin A acid, marketed by Ortho Pharmaceutical Corporation as Retin-A and available by prescription only.

Keep in mind that vitamin E has provoked allergic reactions in some users of cosmetics and treatments containing it.

How to Use Them

I believe that the need for moisturizing lotions and creams has been overstated, at least where normal and oily skin are concerned. But if your skin is dry, you literally cannot overuse moisturizers.

Of course, don't apply any product that upsets your skin by irritating it or triggering an allergic reaction (fragrance and alcohol are among the worst offenders; for other common irritants and allergens, see Chapter 7). And if you're blemish-prone, you should avoid products that contain comedogenic ingredients if possible. (For a list of these, see Chapter 1.) Naturally, if you suspect *any* product of causing problems, stop using it immediately.

Once you find an appropriate product, use it frequently and properly. Otherwise it won't do much good. Here are the moisturizing guidelines I give my patients with dry skin.

• Moisturize immediately after washing and rinsing your face. Towel-blot lightly, then smooth on the product while your skin is still slightly damp. This will "lock in" some of the water remaining after rinsing.

• If it's been more than an hour or so since you last cleansed and moisturized, reapply moisturizer before putting on makeup. The additional moisture will provide a better base for cosmetics and help keep skin well hydrated.

• Apply moisturizer before going outdoors. In warm, humid weather, humectants will draw water from the atmosphere to your skin. When it's cold and windy, the product will minimize moisture loss.

• Before bathing or showering, remove makeup with a light oil or commercial makeup remover, then apply a moisturizer containing humectants. (The steamy warmth will soften skin while humectants attract and hold water vapor.) You can get the same benefits by steaming your face or holding a warm, damp washcloth against it.

Special Care Tips for Dry Facial Skin

Cleansing

I'm a firm believer in soap and water. I don't recommend ordinary brand-name creams or lotions for cleansing even moderately dry skin. Most contain alcohol and soaplike ingredients that are ultimately drying, and do not clean very efficiently unless used in conjunction with a follow-up freshener or toner, which can also be drying. Except in cases of extreme dryness, a mild, superfatted soap or gentle detergent bar is just fine. Basis, Dove, Aveenobar, or any good baby soap are all suitable.

Wash in the morning and before bed. Remove makeup first. Wet your face by splashing with tepid water, then lather up. Do not use a washcloth, complexion brush, or polyester facial sponge; they're too harsh for fragile dry skin. Do not allow suds to stay on your face for more than a minute. Do not relather. Rinse thoroughly with tepid water, blot gently, and apply moisturizer while your skin is still slightly damp.

If your skin is *very* dry and sensitive and you cannot tolerate even a mild soap or detergent bar, try a cleansing lotion such as SFC lotion, Keri Facial Cleanser, Cetaphil Lotion, or pHresh, available at most drugstores. And it might be more comfortable to use a blow-dryer, on the warm (not hot) setting, instead of a towel for drying off. At times when your skin is uncomfortably dry, you may want to think—and *do*—the unthinkable: Skip morning cleansing. If you cleansed thoroughly at bedtime the night before, your face won't be "dirty" when you arise. Simply give it a couple of wake-up splashes of cool water and a dose of moisturizer.

I usually discourage use of a skin toner or freshener for my patients with very dry skin. However, if you like to use one of these follow-up products after cleansing, select one labeled for dry skin. Apply it sparingly, in the morning only, after rinsing your face but before applying moisturizer. If it stings, causes blotches or redness, or seems to make your face dryer, you may have better luck with products formulated for *sensitive* skin. If even these are too harsh, eliminate them from your daily routine, at least for a while. A few weeks of getting more moisture into your skin and your environment (see page 40 for tips on humidifying your home and office)—and/or the arrival of summer, when dryness often lessens—may make it possible for you to resume use of a toner or freshener on a regular basis.

Makeup

Use oil-based cosmetics as opposed to the oil-free kind. They'll act as a further line of defense against moisture loss. Actually, most makeup is oil-based. But the products best suited to dry skin can be identified by words such as "rich," "creamy," "nourishing," and of course "moisturizing" on label or package.

To augment the moisturizing properties of a foundation makeup, pour the amount you expect to use into the palm of your hand, add a dot of moisturizing cream or lotion, and blend with the tip of a finger before you apply it.

If your skin is dry and sensitive, use hypoallergenic or sensitive-skin products. However, keep in mind that even though a product is made with few or none of the most common irritants and allergens, it still might cause a reaction in your skin. If you suspect that something you are putting on your face is causing problems, discontinue use immediately. Take a look at the ingredient list and try another brand made with as many *different* ingredients as possible.

The best advice of all for anyone whose skin is dry is to be lavish with moisturizers and otherwise to do as little as possible to it. Use cleansers sparingly. Avoid toners and fresheners. Exfoliate infrequently and only if your skin is not particularly sensitive.

See a dermatologist if your skin is very dry, or dry and sensitive, and doesn't respond positively to the suggestions offered here. Doctors can't always work miracles, but they can often track down the source of problems and prescribe individualized regimens that can make significant improvements in the way skin looks and feels.

Dryness Below

Let's shift the focus down now, to the expanse of skin that begins at your shoulders and ends with your feet. Much of the time it's out of sight and out of mind—except when there are problems or when suddenly it's summer and more of you is on view. Then, of course, you want to relieve unattractive dryness as quickly as possible.

Parched, Dry, "Lizard" Skin

Even when skin on arms, torso, and legs is so dry it begins to flake and crack, there's a tendency to simply live with it. But

you don't have to. Assuming that simple dryness hasn't progressed to the point where irritation or infection is present,
the following treatment can be used for allover moisturizing.

Sixty-Minute Antidryness Home "Spa"

You'll need complete privacy in the bathroom and the following products and supplies: a big container of inexpensive
grease or oil (Vaseline or Crisco will work; or you can use salad
or baby oil); baking soda or table salt; a bath brush or scrubber
of loofah or sisal; several towels, including a couple of clean
old ones; a rich moisturizing body cream or lotion; a pumice
stone or callus "file."

1. Close the bathroom door and turn on the shower full
force and hot. The object is to duplicate as closely as possible
the warm, humid ambience of a steam bath.
2. When the room is good and steamy, get undressed. Wrap
a towel around your hair. *Do not go into the shower.* Place an old
towel on bathroom stool, chair, or closed toilet lid and another
on the floor underneath, sit down and slather yourself with
plenty of grease or oil. Grease up your face, too, if it's dry, but
not if you are acne-prone.
3. Pour out a handful of baking soda or salt, and, avoiding
your face and neck, rub it over flaky, rough areas of your body
to soften and remove scaly, dry skin. Use baking soda and rub
very gently if your skin tends to be sensitive. Use salt and rub
a bit more vigorously if your skin is not easily irritated.
4. Turn off the shower and fill the tub with moderately
warm, not hot, water. As the tub fills, use an old, clean towel
to wipe off baking soda or salt and excess grease or oil.
5. Settle into the tub and wash with a mild, nondrying soap
substitute, such as Emulave, or a gentle soap, such as Neutrogena Dry Skin Formula Soap. Use a bath brush or sponge on
roughest, scaliest areas. Treat calluses on balls of feet, toes,
heels, etc., with pumice or foot file.
IMPORTANT: This steam-and-slough treatment is for body skin

only. Do not rub salt or use a bath brush or sponge on your neck or face. Wait until you are out of the tub to cleanse these areas.

6. Limit your time in the tub to five minutes. Pat yourself dry with a clean, soft towel, and immediately apply generous amounts of body lotion or cream.

You can use this spa-type treatment every ten days or so. Together with the dos and don'ts included later in this chapter, it should help relieve ordinary dry-skin flakiness and soften sandpapery areas.

Half-Hour Wrap-up

This is another effective and rather unusual way to relieve dryness and flakiness. You'll need a role of transparent plastic wrap, such as Saran Wrap, body cream or lotion, and a heavy, inexpensive lubricant such as Vaseline.

1. Presteam by running hot water in the shower. Bathroom door should be tightly closed so that steam doesn't escape. When bathroom mirror turns cloudy, humidity is 100 percent. *Do not get into the shower.* Take off your clothes and let your skin "drink in" the moisture for five to ten minutes.

2. Adjust shower temperature to lukewarm, get in and wash with nondrying soap or cleanser. Limit time spent in the shower to five minutes. With a soft towel, blot up excess moisture, leaving skin still slightly damp.

3. Apply body lotion all over. Then coat flaky areas on legs, arms, torso, hands, or feet with inexpensive lubricant. Really layer it on. Then cover with plastic wrap. *Of course, you must never use plastic wrap on your face.* (To lock moisture and lubricant into place on feet, pull on an old pair of socks over the plastic wrap. For hands, get into gloves.)

4. Wait half an hour. (Plastic wrap sticks to itself, so you can move around if you like.) Undo the wrap and wipe off excess lubricant.

De-flaking with Wax

Waxes formulated to remove excess hair will also strip away
scaliness, leaving skin free of fuzz as well as flakes. Waxing can
be done by a professional, at a salon, or you can do it yourself.
(For better home waxing, see the tips in Chapter 8.) Either way,
follow up with a moisturizer.

Extremely Dry, Itchy Skin (Xerosis)

Some skin is not simply dry, it's so dry that in dermatology
there is a special name for it: *xerosis*. Though dryness and extreme dryness shade imperceptibly into each other, in xerosis,
skin may be reddened, itchy, and fissured. In some cases, cracks
are deep enough to bleed. There may be crusted-over patches.
Scratching may result in swelling or an oozing discharge.

When ordinary dryness has progressed to xerosis, the treatments described earlier should *not* be used. Until the condition
improves, the skin needs special, gentle care.

Take fewer baths and showers. I advise patients to limit bathing to twice or three times a week, with daily sponging for
underarms and genitals. Dry areas should be given frequent
applications of a cream or lotion made for extremely dry skin.
Use a .05 percent hydrocortisone cream on itching or inflamed
areas. Reapply the cream every four hours throughout the day.

When you do bathe, use lukewarm, not hot, water. Wash with
a very mild soapless cleanser such as Lowila or Aveenobar.
Don't use a scrubber or even a washcloth on raw, tender areas.
Don't linger in the tub. Spend no more than five minutes in
the water, including the time it takes to rinse. Blot dry with a
soft clean towel; don't rub. Then apply a rich body cream or
lotion. I frequently recommend Complex 15, Ever Soft, Aquaderm, Lubriderm, or Eucerin.

Many cases of extreme dryness respond to a simple cutback
on baths and showers plus increased moisturizing. If redness,
itching, scaling, or cracking get worse, consult a dermatologist.

He or she may decide to prescribe a stronger steroid preparation for your skin.

How to Minimize Body Dryness

• Use a rich moisturizing cream or lotion after *every* exposure
to water. This is the golden rule for dry skin. Follow it each
time you take a shower or bath, wash your hands, or otherwise
get wet.

• Keep showers and baths short, and use tepid, not hot water.
An occasional quick steam bath is okay, but avoid saunas. Keep
your hands out of water as much as possible. When you must
immerse them, wear cotton-lined gloves. If your skin is seri-
ously dry, stay out of chlorinated pools and the ocean. (If you
swim to stay fit, switch to another aerobic activity such as walking or bicycling until your skin improves.)

• Don't use antibacterial or acne-fighting soaps or cleansers
on your body. The only exception is when you are treating oily
or pimple-prone areas on your back. For the same reason—
because it's drying—watch out for alcohol in skin-care products.

• Be aware that traces of laundry detergent, whitening agents,
and bleaches left on clothing and bedding after washing can
contribute to discomfort and irritation, especially in winter
when skin is apt to be driest. If you've been using a heavy-duty
detergent, switch to a milder one. Don't use bleach as a matter
of course, but only when necessary. Use less of all laundry
products than amounts suggested on packaging. Limit your exposure to other household chemicals. Wear gloves when you
can't avoid handling them.

• Keep as much of your body as possible under wraps in cold,
blustery weather. Don't go out into the cold without gloves.
Smooth an extra coating of body lotion on your legs before
getting into panty hose; for even more protection against chapping on calves, wear knee socks, leg warmers, or tights over

hose (you can take them off when you reach your destination).
Pull a hat well down over your forehead on raw, windy days,
and wrap a muffler loosely over mouth and cheeks.

• Since sun, too, is drying, wear an oil-based sunscreen on exposed areas of your body on summer outings. If your body skin
is dry, but your face is oily—not uncommon—you'll need a
second, oil-free sunscreen for your face.

• Carry a moisturizer in your handbag when traveling by plane.
Because air in the pressurized jet cabin is *extremely* drying, apply moisturizer at intervals throughout the flight to face, hands,
arms, legs.

• Drink plenty of water—between six and eight glasses a day.
Though "internal" hydration by itself won't prevent or alleviate
dry skin, drinking too little can contribute to the problem.

• Add more moisture to your indoor environment. Air conditioning in summer and overheating in winter both produce
drying effects. (During the heating season, the average American home has a humidity level of between 5 and 15 percent.
That's dryer than the Sahara desert!) To keep more moisture
in your rooms, consider installing a motor-driven humidifier
that works with your heating system. Or use ultrasonic, cold-
water humidifiers in those rooms in which you spend the most
time. (If your work environment is overly dry, one of these
appliances for the office could be a worthwhile beauty and
health investment.) Use the fireplace only on special, festive
occasions.

Place water-filled bowls on or near radiators. Keep a couple
of inches of water in bathtubs and sinks. When you are at home,
put a large kettle of water on the stove and turn the heat on
to keep it simmering. All will release some moisture into the
air.

Some plant varieties are natural moisturizers, "exhaling"
more water than they drink in. They tend to need plenty of
water themselves. Ferns, bamboo, coleus, spathiphyllum, and
papyrus are examples. Use them to boost the humidity index
in your home. Avoid cacti and other varieties that thrive in
arid environments; they're designed by nature to be efficient

at drawing life-giving moisture from dry soil and air and will further dehydrate your rooms.

"Housemaid's" Knees and Elbows

What causes the roughened, sometimes "pebbly" texture and darkened or reddened skin that used to be characterized as "housemaid's" knees? Lack of moisture mainly, with friction playing a secondary role. Sometimes a previous inflammation in the area contributes to the problem. The condition is often duplicated on elbows. It's nothing to worry about, but it's not pretty, either.

"Housemaid's" knees and elbows sometimes respond to gentle exfoliation that removes the topmost layers of dead skin cells, moisturizing, and mild bleaching to counter discoloration.

Five-Point Program for Smoother Knees and Elbows

1. Before bathing or showering, apply a liberal amount of oil, such as baby oil, plain mineral oil, or even salad oil, to knees and elbows.

2. Pour baking soda into the palm of your hand and massage the oiled areas. Don't overdo. Thirty seconds for each knee and elbow is enough.

3. Bathe as usual. Blot off excess water, then smooth a rich body lotion on knees and elbows. To lock in the moisture, wrap loosely with transparent plastic wrap. Leave on overnight if possible.

4. If your skin is unbroken and free of irritation, use a warm- or cold-wax hair remover on rough areas. It will lift off more of the old, dead skin cells that contribute to the grainy texture and expose newer, smoother skin. The best time to wax is after bathing but before moisturizing.

5. Once a week, mix two tablespoons of fresh lemon juice with a tablespoon of baby oil or other oil and apply to discol-

ored areas with a cotton ball. Leave on for about five minutes.
Rinse thoroughly, then apply body lotion. Or use a commercial
bleach or fade cream made for use on skin. These products are
available at well-stocked drugstores. Use according to package
instructions. Discontinue use if irritation occurs. Commercial
skin bleaches often give good results but are not as effective as
bleaching preparations prescribed by a dermatologist.

How *Not* to Treat "Housemaid's" Knees and Elbows

Patients concerned about the color and texture of the skin on
knees and elbows often tell me that they try to self-treat these
areas as they would calluses on their feet, by scrubbing hard
with a pumice or other harsh abrasive. That's not a good idea.
If you compare the roughened skin on your knees with a callus
on the sole of your foot you'll see that the two are very different. The callus is thicker, tougher, and less sensitive than uncallused areas—which is why you can pumice a callus and feel
no pain. The grainy skin on knees and elbows isn't thick or
tough enough to undergo vigorous abrasion without becoming
sore, irritated, redder, and maybe even rougher than before.
Gentle abrasion, lots of moisture, and perhaps bleaching, as
described above, work better.

Millibumps

Sometimes they look like a sprinkling of tiny whiteheads; sometimes these minuscule raised lesions are reddish; occasionally
they're skin-toned. Despite the similarity to an outbreak of mi-
cropimples, the condition is not related to acne or oily skin
but seems to be somewhat more common in patients whose
skin tends to be dry.

Keratosis pilaris, the dermatological term for the tiny bumps,
is caused when old, dead skin cells don't flake off at the surface
but instead adhere to hair follicles just under the skin. I see it

most frequently on upper arms, but it occurs on thighs too. Like "housemaid's" knees, it poses no health problems, but most of my patients who have this condition want to get rid of it.

The at-home treatment is gentle exfoliation, moisturizing, and peeling.

Alternate-Day Plan for Bumps on Arms and Thighs

1. On day one, bathe or shower with your usual soap. Lather affected areas, then loosen and slough away surface cells by massaging gently with a washcloth or polyester facial sponge. Exert just enough pressure to produce a pleasant tingling sensation; too-harsh scrubbing can cause irritation. Rinse thoroughly. Blot away excess water, leaving skin slightly damp, and apply a moisturizing body lotion.

2. On day two, bathe or shower with your usual soap. Then rewash bumpy areas on arms and thighs with one of the special soaps formulated to produce a mild peeling of the skin, such as Fostex Medicated Cleansing Bar. Rinse thoroughly and pat dry.

IMPORTANT: Don't use a peeling soap for allover bathing. The ingredients that make these cleansers effective in stripping off the topmost layers of skin cells also make them too harsh for use on the entire body—especially when skin tends to be dry.

3. Repeat steps 1 and 2 on alternate days. If your skin shows no sign of irritation after four or five days, try combining the treatments each time you bathe, first massaging gently with a polyester sponge, then rewashing with a peeling soap.

You may begin to see an improvement within ten days after starting do-it-yourself exfoliation and peeling. However, if the condition is persistent and bothersome, check with a dermatologist. Topical preparations available only by prescription offer quicker, surer results. For example, I often include Retin-A, the acne medication that removes the debris of dead skin cells and accelerates the growth of new cells, as part of a treatment program for keratosis pilaris. Another method is to use Lac-Hydrin alone or with Retin-A. Lac-Hydrin is a prescription moisturizer that contains 12 percent lactin, a compound that loosens the tightly compacted keratin plugs (old dead skin cells) that cause the problem.

3

Prettier Eyes in a Wink

If you can't read the fine print, get yourself to an ophthalmologist. But if you want to know what to do about puffiness, bags, sags, wrinkles, and other problems affecting the delicate skin surrounding your eyes, you've turned to the right chapter. The treatments and suggestions provided here have been used successfully by many of my patients. They should work for you too.

Temporary Puffiness

Let's start with puffiness of the upper and lower eyelids. It's often a morning problem. I've had patients tell me that on some mornings their eyes are so puffy they can hardly open them. One said she was so self-conscious about her appearance, she wore sunglasses for the first few hours of the day to disguise the problem.

Many people assume that morning puffiness is somehow related to lack of sleep. Actually, too little sleep has practically nothing to do with morning puffiness. In fact, since the kind of puffiness we're concerned with here is usually the result of body fluids accumulating in the eye area overnight, while the sleeper is horizontal, a case could be made for getting less sleep—spending less time in a horizontal position—as a way of minimizing fluid accumulation and hence puffiness. But there are better approaches to the problem.

How to De-puff Morning Eyes

On arising, immediately splash your face several times with very cold water. This will help improve circulation. After splashing, try any of the following.

• "Tap therapy." With a very light touch, and using fingertips only, gently tap puffy areas on upper and lower lids. Gentle tapping seems to encourage fluids to move away from eyes to other parts of the body. Since it's done standing up, the force of gravity becomes an ally, helping to disperse fluids.

• Get one of those gel-filled masks, available in department stores and pharmacies (they're often sold as an aid for easing headaches and sinus congestion). Place it in the refrigerator before you go to bed at night. Position chilled mask over your eyes in the morning.

• If you don't have a mask, chill ordinary teaspoons and place one over each eye.

• Take a clean washcloth, wring it out with ice-cold water, fold into a rectangle, and place on your eyes.

• Moisten teabags in cold water and apply to eyes.

Preventing Puffiness

Here's what I tell patients who are bothered by swollen lids in the morning.

• Sleep in a position that keeps fluid from "pooling" in your eyes. Try sleeping on your back with your head elevated by two or three plump pillows. Better still, if your bed is the adjustable kind, raise the section that supports your head and shoulders. Or place two or three folded blankets under the head end of your mattress. Or raise the end of the bed frame with a couple of thick planks of wood.

• Reduce fluid intake at bedtime. If you're in the habit of drinking a glass of water, juice, or milk before turning in, stop for a few days and see if your eyes are less puffy in the mornings.

• Salt and foods high in sodium can cause excessive fluid retention. Since so many of us tend to get more dietary salt and sodium than is good for us, a cutback would be a step in the right direction for health and beauty reasons.

• Some eye creams seem to promote puffiness, and occasionally a rash, in certain women. If you've been wearing eye cream to bed, try applying a bit less or use a cream or lotion with a lighter texture. Instead of smoothing it on the entire eye area, keep it at least one-quarter inch away from lower lashes and dot it on the upper lid from brow to crease only.

If a change in application technique doesn't help, you may be allergic or sensitive to something in the cream. Check ingredients on the label against the list of common allergens and irritants on page 125. Another possibility is that the cream you are using is doing its job *too* well and that in plumping up wrinkles, it's also puffing up the surrounding eye area. See what happens when you skip the cream for a night or two.

Improvement after a few nights without eye cream does not necessarily mean that you should never wear one of these products. However, it's a pretty good indication that you should switch to a different one. As a general rule, the heaviest, oiliest formulations are most apt to contribute to puffiness. Why not experiment with some of the lighter ones that list water as the first ingredient on the label? Eye gels are another possibility, since most of them are even lighter in texture than creams.

• Puffiness can also be the result of a cold or an allergy to dust, pollen, animal hair, etc., in which case an over-the-counter medication formulated to relieve cold and allergy symptoms, such as Dristan, Allerest, or Chlor-Trimeton, might help. In considering what you might be allergic to, keep in mind that allergies to down and feathers are not uncommon. (One patient's puffiness improved dramatically in summer when she packed away the expensive down comforter she'd been sleeping with during the cold-weather months.)

Cosmetic Camouflage

The above suggestions can help relieve puffiness. Makeup can camouflage it or even make it disappear.

To minimize upper-lid puffiness with makeup, you'll need two eye shadow colors, a medium shade and lighter one in the same family. Taupe and pale beige, for example, or a medium blue and a lighter blue.

NOTE: If your skin is smooth, unwrinkled, and normal to oily, you can wear powder or cream shadow. If it's dry and the area above your eyelids is visibly aged, cream shadows are a better choice. Though they require a bit more blending than powder formulations to achieve a natural look, creams are better for your skin, tend to last longer, and downplay crepiness on lids.

1. Apply the darker shade to your entire upper lid, from just below the brow to lashes. Blend carefully with fingertip or applicator. What you want is an even "wash" of neutral color. This darker hue will act as a kind of base coat for the lighter one.

2. With a clean applicator or finger, stroke the lighter shade on bottom half of upper lid, from crease to lashes. With lower portion of lid highlighted, the puffiness is less apparent.

Puffiness, or bags, under the eyes requires a different approach. Don't stroke on a concealer lighter in color than your skin tone or foundation makeup. Pale shades seem to come forward and catch the eye, so a light-toned concealer will only make bags seem more pronounced. Instead, use your regular foundation and a second, slightly darker one in the same color family. If the only darker shade you can find is a lot darker, lighten it with a dot of your regular shade. For the procedure that follows, too much contrast is worse than too little.

1. Apply regular foundation as usual, dotting and blending it over your entire face, including the bags.
2. With the tip of your finger, place two or three dots of the darker foundation on bags only. Blend carefully, so that there are no obvious lines of demarcation.

Permanent Puffiness

Sooner or later, depending on your genes, your health, your habits, and the way you care for your skin, a certain amount of "puffiness" may become permanent. As years go by, the delicate, thin skin around the eyes becomes even thinner and less elastic and the layer of muscles underlying it begins to thin and stretch. Fatty tissue surrounding the eyes, tissue which in youth is held firmly in place by those muscles, eventually pushes through. The result is the heavy, sagging upper lid and baggy lower lid associated with age. When that happens, fluid accumulation can add to the problem, but it's no longer a primary cause.

Cosmetic camouflage can help make even permanent sags and bags less obvious, but nothing short of cosmetic surgery will take away the puffiness. If it *really* bothers you, you might want to consider one of the procedures developed to tighten and smooth upper and lower lids. The name for this type of surgery is *blepheraoplasty*.

Crow's-feet and Other Eye Lines

As you'll soon see, there are several things you can do to forestall the appearance of fine lines around your eyes. But sooner or later, we all begin to see fine lines that weren't there when we were younger. Here's a trick for making very fine lines in the eye area less noticeable:

1. Wash your face as usual. Apply a moisturizer if you ordinarily wear one.
2. Beat the white of an egg until it's frothy.
3. With a clean, fine-pointed makeup brush, the kind used with liquid eyeliner, "paint" egg white into the lines.
4. Wait three or four minutes, or until the egg white is dry.
5. Proceed with your usual makeup.

Though results are short-lived, the egg-white treatment tends to tighten the area and, used under foundation, "plasters over" tiny lines, helping to hide them.

I've noticed a couple of commercial products that work on the same principle. One is called Line Fill, by Adrien Arpel.

Not only is the skin around your eyes very thin and delicate, it's also not as well supplied with oil glands as the rest of the face. In addition, eyes are active. They're in constant motion. They crinkle up in a smile. They open wide in surprise. They squeeze closed to hold back tears and for protection in a brisk wind. They squint shut in bright light. It's no wonder that this fragile, relatively dry skin, subject to so much stretching and compressing, is the first on the body to show signs of aging. That's a fact. But it's also a fact that at least some "aging" is self-inflicted.

Recently a woman I'll call Catherine came to my office to discuss having a mole removed. She was a new patient, I'd never seen her before, and at first glance I supposed her to be in her late thirties, possibly early forties. Wrong! According to the preliminary information my nurse had taken from her, Catherine was thirty-one years old. I'm rarely that far off in judging a person's age, so I took a closer look and saw why I'd been mistaken. Though her face was basically firm and smooth, the skin around her eyes was creased and wrinkled enough to make her look almost a decade older than she was.

Why would someone so young have such noticeable wrinkling? I didn't try to find out. After all, she was there to see me about a completely different matter and unless she mentioned the lines around her eyes, I had to assume she wasn't concerned about them. (The last thing I want to do is create a problem that doesn't exist.) But it was hard for me not to get up on my soapbox, because I'm convinced her wrinkles weren't inevitable. Thirty-one-year-old skin around the eyes shouldn't look like that. With good commonsense care, even forty-five-year-old skin can be smooth and relatively unlined.

Don't skip the information that follows. There's a lot you can do to forestall aging of the skin around the eyes, no matter what your age now.

• Buy a good pair of polarized or anti-ultraviolet sunglasses and wear them on sunny days year-round. Squinting is a reflex action beyond your conscious control, and this involuntary bunching up of the muscles around the eyes is a cause of early wrinkling.

• Don't smoke. Squinting through the fumes also tends to create deeper wrinkles around the eyes at an earlier age. There are dozens of other more important reasons not to smoke, of course. This is just one more to add to the list.

• Don't do facial exercises. I'm always amazed when some so-called expert, who should know better, recommends them. Though it's true that muscles around the eyes weaken with age, there is no evidence to indicate that facial workouts strengthen those muscles and prevent wrinkles and sagging. On the contrary, winking, popping your eyes, arching your eyebrows, grimacing, and other facial calisthenics can accelerate the transformation of tiny expression lines into wrinkles.

• To avoid unnecessary stretching of the skin, don't touch the area around your eyes any more than you have to. When you must touch, do it gently. Use a very light tapping, dabbing, or blotting motion. Do not rub.

• Don't use cosmetics so heavy or dense in texture that they must be dragged across the eye area. Products to be used on the lids should glide on. For this reason, many stick-type concealers are less desirable than creams or liquids. Before you buy, test cream or pencil eye shadow on your wrist to make sure color slides on easily, with no tugging. Powder shadows are easier to apply, but some need to be rubbed in for an evenly blended look. Again, test before you buy.

• Remove eye makeup as gently as you put it on. You can use a commercial product (I often suggest Andrea Eye-Q pads, which come in two formulas, oil-base and nonoily, for my patients who wear contact lenses) or a light oil, such as baby oil or vegetable oil, for this purpose. Some of my patients prefer a liquifying cream, such as Albolene.

To remove mascara with oil: Pour a small amount of oil onto a clean cotton ball. Press out the excess. With your free hand, hold a tissue under lashes and with the other hand, wipe lashes from base to tips with the oiled cotton ball. Wipe again with a fresh, clean cotton ball. Repeat, alternating oiled and fresh cotton until the fresh one comes away clean.

Follow instructions on the label when using a commercial eye makeup remover, always being careful not to pull or stretch your lids as you work.

• Even if the skin on the rest of your face is fairly oily, lubricate the area around your eyes. (Remember, lids are not well endowed with oil glands.) Almost every major cosmetics company makes at least one eye cream or gel. Some are fragrance-free and/or hypoallergenic. Some are meant to be used at bedtime only; others can be worn overnight and during the day under makeup. (Many of the latter contain sunscreening ingredients, which provide essential protection.) I know a few models who can afford the most expensive eye creams but prefer to dab on a small amount of Vaseline at night. Another model, one of my patients, likes to use—are you ready for this?—Preparation H. Yes, the over-the-counter product for relief of hemorrhoids. She likes the texture.

However, it would be a mistake to assume that *any* lubricant or moisturizer is a good substitute for eye cream. Some face, hand, and body creams are not suitable because they're made

with ingredients that are relatively safe to use elsewhere but
that might irritate sensitive skin around the eyes. (Most of these
ingredients are purposely omitted from creams developed for
use in the eye area.) Face, hand, and body *lotions*—even those
free of potential eye irritants—are poor choices because they
are essentially liquids and don't stay put unless rubbed in. For
the same reason, creams that liquify at skin temperature are
not suitable for overnight use on the eyes.

• To minimize sun-related wrinkling and other damage, don't
go out without first applying a sunscreen that is labeled safe
for use in the eye area. I can't emphasize enough the impor-
tance of sun protection for everyone, throughout the year, not
just in the eye area but on all exposed skin. (For more about
sun protection, see Chapter 9.)

Dark Circles

There are almost as many reasons for undereye circles as there
are complaints about them, but the main reason has to do with
the fact that skin under the eyes is thin. It's so thin in some
people that blood passing through the tiny veins near the surface shows through, giving the area a bluish or grayish cast. As
a general rule, the thinner and more transparent your skin, the
greater the contrast between the area under the eyes and other
areas. The pallor that often accompanies fatigue, a cold, or
other ailment can accentuate the difference, which explains
why, when you're tired or feeling under the weather, undereye
circles are more pronounced.

In some people, undereye circles tend to be brownish and
permanent. This may be due to hyperpigmentation—the presence of greater than usual amounts of melanin, which gives
skin its color.

Whatever the cause or the color, though, cosmetics can provide a solution.

How to Lighten Up Dark Circles in Five Minutes or Less

1. After moisturizing, but before applying foundation, dot undereye area with a color-correcting underbase. (These products are just what their name implies. Worn under foundation, they counteract unwanted skin tones. A pale green color corrector makes red skin look less ruddy; pale pink warms up sallow skin; etc.) If circles are bluish, counteract with a pale yellow underbase. For brown circles, try pale blue or mauve. Blend underbase on undereye area only. Use your fingertip or a damp sponge.

2. Allow a minute or two for underbase to dry, then apply foundation in a shade close to your natural skin tone.

3. With a soft makeup brush or clean puff, apply loose powder over your entire face. Then "set" it by patting gently with a slightly damp sponge.

NOTE: Until you find the right underbase, you can tone out circles with concealer. Avoid using very pale, almost white, concealer. Best results are achieved with one that is only slightly lighter than your foundation. One of my patients who is a makeup artist says you can make your own custom-blended concealer—not too light, not too dark—by mixing a dot of moisturizer into a drop or two of foundation. Correct the color if necessary, by blending in a bit more of either.

If you are healthy, get enough sleep, eat properly, exercise moderately, and you are not unduly stressed, yet you *still* have dark circles, they are probably there to stay. Self-treatment begins and ends with cosmetic camouflage. Perfect your technique.

If you want to go a step further, consult a dermatologist. In some cases, special prescription bleaching creams, Retin-A, and perhaps an in-office chemical peel, which removes topmost layers of the skin, can result in noticeable improvement. *Don't look for instant improvement.* It takes some time for bleaching and Retin-A to work, and chemical peels may have to be repeated before results are visible.

Red, Irritated Eyes

Whether they're the result of a cold or allergy, too much wind and sun, a good cry, or of using cosmetics that irritate, they're an eyesore.

Fifteen-Minute Treatment to Refresh Red, Swollen, Teary Eyes

1. Try eyedrops formulated to relieve allergy and cold symptoms, such as Visine or Murine. But before you even open the bottle, double check that what you are about to put in your eye is indeed eyedrops. You can never be too careful; mistakes can cause injury or blindness. Be sure to use drops according to instructions on the label.

IMPORTANT: Don't make a habit of treating your eyes with drops containing vasoconstrictors (which constrict blood vessels in the eyes) and antihistamines. Check labels to see if they warn against frequent use. Used too often, these products tend to become less and less effective and in some cases eventually contribute to red-eye syndrome.

2. While the eyedrops are working, apply one of the following to your lids: a clean cloth wrung out of cold water; cold, damp tea bags; chilled cucumber or potato slices; or a commercial product such as Elizabeth Arden Puffiness Calming Eye Gel. You should apply these while lying down or sitting back in a comfortable chair for five minutes or so.

3. Apply foundation or concealer slightly lighter than your natural skin tone to counteract lingering redness. A dot of concealer blended just under the highest point of the eyebrow arch can make eyes look fresher and clearer.

4. Try blue eyeliner. It will make the white of your eyes seem brighter. (Skip the liner, however, if your lids still feel irritated.)

Eye Makeup Safety Tips

If your eyes are irritated, cosmetics may be to blame. Tearing, redness, itching, or stinging can be caused by using the wrong makeup, or the right makeup in the wrong way. The following guidelines could help prevent future problems.

• If you are allergy-prone, use hypoallergenic products. These contain less or none of the most common, known allergens and irritants. Keep in mind, though, that the term "hypoallergenic" is not a guarantee of anything. It may be that the skin around your eyes is too sensitive even for some of these products. If problems develop, experiment with different brands of mascara, shadow, liner, et cetera, always giving your eyes a two- or three-day vacation from makeup between tryouts. Dispose of any cosmetics that cause irritation so you won't be tempted to use them again. If problems persist, discontinue use of all eye makeup and see a doctor.

• Neither borrow nor lend eye makeup. This applies whether or not your eyes are sensitive or allergy-prone. Microorganisms that cause irritation or infection can be spread via eye makeup.

• Don't use store test products on your eyes. It's extremely risky. When deciding which brand and color to buy, stroke the test product on the inside of your wrists. To gauge whether the color works with your eyes and skin, hold your wrist up close to your face.

• Don't use any product not specifically formulated for eyes on your eyes. Because of FDA regulations, ingredients in eye makeup are generally safer and less likely to irritate than ingredients used in cosmetics meant to be applied to other areas of the face.

• Throw out unused mascara after four months. Get rid of unused shadows, liners, concealers, and other eye makeup after a year. Because eyes are so sensitive, the high-powered preservatives commonly used in other cosmetics are omitted from eye makeup; thus it deteriorates and becomes susceptible to contamination more rapidly than those other cosmetics. Since heat accelerates deterioration, don't take eye makeup to the

beach, leave it on hot, sunny windowsills or in the glove com-
partment of your car in summer.

• Whenever possible, use your clean fingertips or disposable
applicators, such as cotton balls and Q-tips, to apply eye
makeup. When using a brush or sponge, make sure it's clean
by washing it in sudsy warm water.

• If you've had problems with mascara, try applying it to lash
tips only. Unless your lashes are very short and sparse, avoid
using "lash extender" mascaras; the tiny fibers in these mascaras are potential troublemakers for contact lens wearers and
those whose eyes are very sensitive. As a general rule, cake
mascara is less irritating than other kinds.

• Eyeliner pencils seem to cause fewer problems than liquid
and powder shadows. The safest way to line your eyes is to
stroke color just above the lashes on your upper lid and *below*
the lashes on your lower lid. Conjunctivitis and other problems
can result from lining along the pink rim of your lower lid
above the lashes. Don't moisten the point of the pencil with
the tip of your tongue in an attempt to soften it. (To do so
might transfer microorganisms in saliva to your eyes.) If a pencil is too hard for easy color application, a tiny bit of petroleum
jelly on the point will help color go on smoothly.

• Some iridescent, pearlized, or frosted eye shadow formulations are more likely to irritate than matte-finish shadows. Keep
this in mind if your eyes are very sensitive.

• Nail polish—or rather, the fumes released from fresh polish
on nails—can cause tearing and a stinging sensation if wafted
too near eyes. For this reason, don't apply polish immediately
before making up eyes. And if your eyes are easily irritated,
make sure the room is well ventilated when you use polish.

Lash Disaster

One day you look in the mirror and see just a few skimpy
spikes where your lashes used to be. What's the problem? Probably nothing serious.

Just rubbing your eyes a lot can cause eyelash breakage and

fallout. So can improper mascara removal. Or perhaps the growth cycle is somewhat out of sync.

Hair, including the hair on your head, body hair, eyebrows, and eyelashes, grows in cycles. An eyelash, for example, grows for about six months, then goes into a resting phase and finally drops out or is pushed out by a new lash developing in the follicle. Cycles tend to overlap, so that as old hairs are lost, other hairs are reaching maturity, and the number of full-grown lashes on your lids remains approximately the same. But occasionally, an unusually large number of lashes will reach the resting stage and fall out at about the same time.

Give eyes and lashes extra gentle treatment, and you'll probably see noticeable growth in a month or so. If there's no improvement, see a dermatologist; there may be a problem he or she can help you with.

How to Have Longer, Thicker Eyelashes in Six Minutes

1. Use a roll-on mascara, the kind with an applicator brush that screws into its own tubelike dispenser, or cake mascara, which is sold with its own separate brush. Load brush with plenty of mascara and stroke through tops of upper lashes, coating them from base to ends. (It's easier if your lids are half-closed.)

2. Reload the brush, and with eyes wide open, coat undersides of upper lashes.

3. Coat ends of upper lashes by moving the brush horizontally across the tips.

4. With a clean cotton ball, apply a *light* dusting of face powder to upper lashes, then separate them with a tiny eyelash comb. An old, clean cake mascara brush can be used to separate if you don't have an eyelash comb.

TIP: Since applying mascara is one of the last steps in your makeup routine, you may want to use a clean tissue to protect the area directly under your eyes from mascara speckles. With your free hand, hold the tissue under the eye you are working on.

5. Reload the brush and stroke mascara on tops of lower lashes, from base to tips.

6. Coat ends of bottom lashes by moving the brush horizontally across the tips, then separate them to avoid clumping.

7. Repeat steps 1 through 3, and comb through upper lashes to separate. For even thicker, longer-looking lashes, powder again and apply a third coat.

TIP: Curled lashes "open up" the eyes and help make them look bigger and more wide-awake. But if you use an eyelash curler, do it before you apply mascara. In curling afterward, you run the risk of smudging your handiwork. Also, not-quite-dry mascaraed lashes may adhere to the curler and be pulled out.

Eyebrow Tweezer Twinge

Brows look neater after you've reshaped them and plucked out the strays. But the process can leave the area pink and sore.

Here's how to minimize tweezer twinge in three minutes:

1. Immediately after tweezing, apply ice-cold cloth compresses or crushed ice in a plastic sandwich bag. Hold in place for about a minute.

2. Dampen a cotton ball with a gentle astringent, such as witch hazel, and dab on tweezed areas.

3. Pat dry with a clean towel, then smooth on a light moisturizer.

4. Wait at least half an hour before applying makeup.

This quick treatment should take away most of the sting and get reddened skin quickly back to normal. Nevertheless, it's always best to shape brows in the evening after bath or shower so that by morning any trace of irritation will be gone.

Safe and Easy Brow Shaping

Occasionally a patient will come in with an inflammation in the eyebrow area, the result of careless tweezing. I can't promise that the following method will prevent such problems, but it will reduce the risk, as well as some of the discomfort, of plucking.

1. Remove eye makeup and wash your face.
2. Saturate a cotton ball with rubbing alcohol, press out the excess, and wipe it across the length of each eyebrow and on any strays you want to get rid of. (Alcohol will clean the areas and remove traces of oil that might prevent tweezers from getting a firm grip on hairs.) Give tweezers an alcohol wipe too.
3. Hold over your brows a washcloth that has been soaked in very warm water and wrung out. Heat opens pores and should make it easier to pull hairs from their follicles.
4. Starting with strays between your brows, tweeze one hair at a time, always working in the direction of hair growth—*away* from the nose in most cases, though between-brow hairs often grow straight up.
5. Get a good grip on base of hair as close to the skin as possible (this is easier if you use your free hand to gently stretch the skin near your hair). Pluck it out with a quick, *decisive* pull.

TIP: If plucking *hurts*, try applying an ice cube to the area you're working on. The cold will close pores, but it will also have a numbing effect.

6. Shape brows from underside only. Unless you have the patience, fortitude, and time for frequent redos, don't make exaggerated changes in their length or thickness. However, a few *minor* corrections can make an attractive difference in your looks.

For example:

To create the illusion of wide-set eyes and/or a slimmer nose, tweeze inner ends of brows so that they begin just beyond the inner corners of your eyes.

To make very wide-set eyes appear closer together, narrow

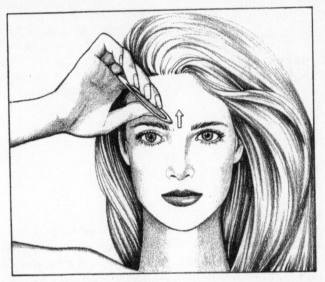

To shape brows, tweeze in the direction of hair growth. If strays between the brows grow up, for example, tweeze them in an upward direction, as shown.

the distance between brows by penciling in a few "hairs" at inner ends.

To give your whole face a youthful "lift," shorten outer ends of brows to achieve a subtle "upswept" or winged look.

7. Instead of thinning very bushy brows by tweezing, brush the hairs straight down and trim along the natural arch with manicure scissors. Then brush up and out.

Discipline for Unruly Brows

If eyebrow hairs tend to curl or point down when you want them to go up and out, you can "set" them with hair-setting gel. Place a dot on an eyebrow brush or an old clean tooth-brush, then comb through brows in the desired direction.

4

Liptricks

As every dermatologist knows, there's a wide range of conditions that are special to the lips and the skin surrounding them. From cold sores to chapping, from cheilitis (I'll tell you what *that* is later in this chapter) to crinkles and cracks, here are my recommendations for dealing with those problems and for making sure your mouth always says nice things about you.

Cold Sores (Herpes Labialis)

They begin with itching, tingling, and a "drawing" sensation, then gradually redden and erupt into a painful blister or cluster of blisters. They are sometimes called fever blisters. Usually they heal without treatment within a week or so, but while they last, they're uncomfortable and can be unattractive. Here's what I tell patients who want to know how to reduce the discomfort and perhaps speed up the healing process.

1. As soon as you become aware of the itching or tingling sensation of a cold sore in the making, apply ice. (Crush one or two cubes, place them in a plastic sandwich bag, and hold the bag against your lip for ten minutes.) Repeat several times a day if possible.

2. After each application of ice, dot on a small amount of

Resolve, a gel-type medication containing anesthetic ingredients, sold over the counter at most pharmacies. Resolve and similar medications are most effective in combating cold sores when their use is begun in the pre-blister stage.

3. To dry up blisters and encourage quicker healing, dab them with a cotton swab saturated in Listerine. Or apply compresses of sterile gauze soaked with cold Burow's Solution. You can mix up your *own* solution by dissolving two tablets or two packets of Domeboro, which is available at pharmacies, in a pint of cold water. Use in this strength until blisters begin to dry. Thereafter, to avoid overdrying the lips, apply a weaker solution of one packet or one tablet per pint of cold water. Confine soaks to cold sores only, avoiding unaffected areas of the mouth and lips.

Dispose of cotton swabs and gauze pads immediately after use.

4. Allow dried, blistered skin to fall off by itself. Picking or peeling could lead to a secondary infection, and possibly to scarring.

Cold Sore Dos and Don'ts

• Don't touch a cold sore except when treating it as above. To lessen the risk of infection, wash your hands before administering home treatments and medication. Wash again afterward to avoid spreading the cold sore virus to other parts of your body, especially the eyes. A herpes infection near the eye should be seen immediately by a doctor; it could lead to blindness. The herpes virus, which causes cold sores, is highly contagious, so avoid kissing and other close physical contact until blisters are no longer visible. (The virus responsible for cold sores, *herpes labialis*, also called *herpes simplex I*, can be spread by hand or mouth to the genital area. Genital herpes, or *herpes simplex II*, can be transferred in the same way to the mouth.)

• Don't wear lipstick until blistered areas have healed. Bacteria present in the lipstick can lead to a secondary infection. In addition, manipulation of the area as lip color is applied could slow the healing process.

If you want to wear something on your mouth, try a little Blistex or other lip lubricant. It won't add color but will give a nice shine, and because it slides on more easily than lipstick, it shouldn't interfere with healing.

• Don't apply hydrocortisone products to cold sores. The steroids in these medications can encourage spreading of the virus.

• Do protect your mouth and lips from ultraviolet rays, which can activate the cold sore virus. One of my patients, a dedicated sun worshiper, used to get the lesions as often as twice a month in summer, but for a long time she ignored suggestions to stay out of the sun or wear a lipstick or other lip product with built-in sun protection. It took a nasty infection and minor scarring to convince her to take precautions. They seem to have helped; she has far fewer cold sores now.

• Do take measures to prevent the chapped, dry condition that makes lips more vulnerable to the cold sore virus. Wear a lip lubricant or conditioner, or a creamy, moisturizing lipstick indoors and out, day and night, especially in winter.

• Do check with a dermatologist if cold sores ooze a honey-colored fluid that dries to an amber crust. This often signals the presence of secondary, bacterial infection.

• Finally, if you are plagued with frequent cold sores, consult your dermatologist. He or she may want to prescribe a new drug, acyclovir, that, if taken regularly, might shorten the duration of active infection and help prevent recurrences.

Dry, Chapped Lips

Extreme dryness and chapping is usually a cold weather problem, but some of my patients who sail, jog, or play a lot of tennis or golf develop the condition in summer too. The best way to deal with chapped lips is as follows:

1. Smear a thick coating of petroleum jelly on your lips. Cover with a washcloth or other clean cloth wrung out of very warm water. Hold the cloth against your lips for several minutes.

2. With a fresh cloth wrung out of very warm water, gently

massage petroleum jelly into your lips. Keep the cloth warm by dunking and wringing again as soon as it begins to cool. Continue massaging until most of the petroleum jelly has been absorbed.

3. Blot your mouth and immediately apply a lip lubricant or conditioner. If you are going outdoors, use one with sunscreening ingredients.

How to Prevent Dryness and Chapping

• Habitual lip licking is the single most common cause of chapped lips, in both summer and winter. Each time you run your tongue over your lips, you wet them. The moisture quickly evaporates, causing lips to feel dry. You lick again to remoisten, and post-evaporation dehydration makes your lips feel drier still. The result, finally, can be a reddened, sore mouth with very dry, flaky, even cracked lips.

It's not easy to stop licking, especially if you do it without thinking. One way to control it, though, is to suck on a sugar-free sour ball or other hard candy. This tip has helped several of my patients break the habit. Try it. With a sourball in your mouth, it's almost impossible to run your tongue over your lips.

• Wear petroleum jelly or a lip conditioner overnight.

• Don't allow astringents, toners, skin fresheners, and other products containing alcohol, which of course is very drying, to come into contact with your lips. Avoid your mouth when using a facial scrub, mask, or grains. Be especially careful with benzoyl peroxide and other anti-acne products, including Retin-A. All of these are formulated to dry and peel the skin, and that's what they'll do to your lips.

• Choose lipsticks made with a high concentration of emollient ingredients. They can be identified by key words in ads and on packaging, words such as "rich," "creamy," and "moisturizing." Most of these are formulated with a higher percentage of protective oils and waxes than lipsticks advertised as being "long-lasting."

• Since dry indoor air during the heating season can aggravate chapping, try to get more moisture into your home or office. You'll find a number of suggestions for humidifying your surroundings in Chapter 2.

Hot Lips (Cheilitis)

Inflammation and swelling, with or without flaking or cracking, point to a condition known as *cheilitis*. I've called it "hot lips" here, because it's frequently accompanied by an uncomfortable burning sensation.

I seem to be seeing more cheilitis in women now than a few years ago. The increase, I suspect, has something to do with the rise in adult acne and the use of drying anti-acne medications.

Myra is typical in this regard. After years of trouble-free skin, she began to break out when she was in her middle thirties. For her, cheilitis was partly the result of misusing Retin-A, which had been prescribed to fight her acne. She misused it by applying too much, and instead of following instructions to keep the Retin-A from coming into contact with her lips, she carelessly smeared it over her entire mouth. Lip licking and going out into the sun without a sun block or sunscreen compounded the problem.

Most cases of cheilitis, however, are the outcome of contact with other irritants or allergens. When an allergen is involved, there may also be a crop of rashlike blisters. *Actinic cheilitis*, on the other hand, is activated by sun exposure. Whatever the cause, cheilitis is more likely to occur when lips are in a parched, chapped state.

Do-It-Yourself Relief from Cheilitis

1. Wash the area with a gentle soap and lukewarm water. Rinse and pat dry with a clean, soft towel.
2. Apply ice—crushed and placed in a plastic bag—to re-

duce burning and ease swelling and itching. (Or, if you have one in the house, use a well-chilled gel-type thermal pack.) To protect your mouth from excessive cold, place a folded tissue or thin, clean cloth between lips and ice-filled bag or thermal pack, then gently hold in position for several minutes.

3. Smooth on a film of over-the-counter 0.5 percent hydrocortisone ointment such as Cortaid or Caldecort. This should further minimize discomfort and swelling.

4. Wait a couple of hours after applying hydrocortisone, then dab on a lip lubricant containing sunscreening ingredients, such as Blistex Daily Conditioning Treatment for Lips.

5. Alternate applications of hydrocortisone ointment and lip lubricant throughout the day. Use more ice when convenient or necessary to ease burning and swelling.

6. Do not wear lipstick or gloss, and don't line your lips with pencil until inflammation and swelling have subsided and your mouth is back to normal.

Preventive Measures for Cheilitis

First, I want to reiterate that dry, chapped lips are more vulnerable to cheilitis, and the most important preventive measures are those that keep your mouth in good condition. The antichapping guidelines on pages 65–66 will help.

But though dryness and chapping make your lips more susceptible, there are almost always additional factors involved. Your answers to the following questions should help you (and your dermatologist, if you need one) track down the causes so that you can guard against the cheilitis in the future.

• Is the condition more severe on your lower lip? If so, it may be actinic cheilitis, which is activated by sunlight. Actinic cheilitis should be treated by a dermatologist. Make an appointment, and in the meantime self-treat as explained above. Don't leave the house without first applying sun protection to your lips.

• Is inflammation greatest along the edges of your mouth, where facial skin and lip skin meet? And if so, have you been using a lip pencil to line your mouth before filling in with lipstick? Two yesses may mean that you are sensitive or allergic to one or more ingredients in the pencil—probably one of the dyes. Stop lining your lips for a few weeks. When you resume, use a hypoallergenic brand and see what happens.

• Are exposed surfaces of both lips equally affected? The problem could be your lipstick or gloss. Trouble can arise immediately after the first wearing of a new product, or flare up suddenly after weeks or months of using an old standby. Certain dyes, particularly D & C Red #21 and #27, are thought to be a factor leading to cheilitis in a small percentage of women. Fragrance is a fairly common allergen. Other ingredients in lip-coloring products that have caused problems in the allergy-prone are lanolin, castor oil, beeswax, carnauba wax, antioxidants, and alcohol. If you suspect a connection between cheilitis and lipstick, stop wearing it for a while. Then try one of the hypoallergenic brands.

• Are soreness, burning, and swelling most pronounced on inner areas where lip meets lip? This could indicate sensitivity to any of a wide variety of foods, though in my experience, mangoes, citrus fruits, and artichokes are the most common offenders. Naturally, if your lips puff up and feel hot after eating something out of the ordinary, avoid that food in the future.

• Cheilitis could also be a reaction to certain ingredients in nail polish. (It takes hours for polish to cure—that is, dry completely. Until then, if you happen to be sensitive or allergic to something in the product, touching your mouth with newly polished nails, even if they feel dry, could trigger the condition.) When a flare-up occurs soon after a manicure, remove the polish, and wait a week or so to see what happens. Next time you do your nails, try a hypoallergenic product.

• In some cases, nickel appears to be the instigator. Do you use your teeth to open bobby pins or paper clips? Is your lipstick so worn down that the metal container comes into contact with your mouth when you apply it? Since nickel is an ingredient in many common, everyday containers, utensils, and gadgets, it's hard to avoid. But make the effort if you suspect it as a cause of cheilitis.

What if none of the above seem to apply, and the condition persists despite home treatment? You know the answer: Consult a dermatologist. He or she can prescribe stronger medications to reduce discomfort and swelling. And through careful questioning, and perhaps testing for allergies and sensitivities, your doctor should be able to determine which substances and/or practices are making a mess of your mouth.

"Cracked" Corners (Perleche)

Soreness, inflammation, and cracked skin at the *corners* of the mouth are signs of a condition known as *perleche*. It's most common in people with a tendency to drool—the very young, usually, and the very old. But it's not confined to these two age extremes. Under certain circumstances it can affect almost anyone. When it does, it's uncomfortable and unattractive, since redness and cracking often extend well below the lower corners of the mouth, affecting skin in the chin area and giving the mouth an unpleasant, turned-down expression.

Some of my patients with perleche have had good results with what I call "triple-layer" therapy, which encourages healing and helps reduce some of the discomfort associated with the condition:

1. Wash your face, rinse thoroughly, and pat dry.
2. Dot an over-the-counter fungicide, such as Monistat cream, on affected areas. (Perleche is caused in part by a yeastlike fungus thriving in moisture at the corners of the mouth.)
3. Dab a small amount of over-the-counter 0.5 percent hydrocortisone cream over the fungicide. This will soothe some of the soreness.
4. Top it all off with a thin film of antibacterial ointment such as Polysporin or Bacitracin.

5. Repeat three times a day—four would be even better, if you can manage it. If you start on a Friday morning, you should see some improvement by Monday.

What about lipstick? I tell patients not to wear it until the condition is pretty much cleared up, since ingredients in the product might irritate and complicate the problem. On the special occasions when you feel you *must* wear a little lipstick, apply it so that color stops short of the reddened, cracked corners of your mouth.

Preventing Perleche

There's no guarantee you'll never have a relapse, but the condition will be less likely to return if you take these precautions:

• Keep lips well lubricated and protected against chapping. The micoorganisms that contribute to perleche have a better chance of taking hold when skin is irritated.
• Make sure your diet is adequate. Faulty nutrition, especially a deficiency of vitamin B_2, is sometimes a factor in the development of perleche. Good food sources of B_2 are green vegetables, such as broccoli and spinach, and dairy products, such as milk and yogurt. If there is some reason that you might not be able to get enough B_2 and other essential nutrients from food, consider taking a multivitamin and mineral supplement. Be careful to get enough but not too much vitamin A and E, because excessive amounts of these can make lips more vulnerable to chapping.
• Correct a malocclusion (poor alignment of teeth in upper and lower jaws), which can distort the mouth and lips in ways that encourage saliva buildup in the corners. The chapping that results increases susceptibility to perleche. Your dentist has probably told you already if you have a "bad bite." Correcting it will be good for your teeth, good for your looks, and perhaps put an end to a problem with perleche.

Mango Sensitivity

A month or so ago, a woman came to see me about redness, swelling, and blisters around her mouth. The area was extremely itchy, and the skin on her upper lip was peeling and raw from scratching. The condition didn't look like any of the problems that commonly affect the mouth. In fact, more than anything else, it looked like poison ivy.

I asked her what had happened. She said she didn't know; she couldn't figure it out. Had she recently eaten anything unusual? I prompted. After thinking a moment, she told me she'd had a fruit salad, made with mangoes, at a luncheon on the day the problem first appeared. Then it all fell into place.

Mango resins are chemically similar to poison ivy resins, and people who are sensitive to the latter can experience a poison-ivy-like reaction when they eat a mango. Fortunately, the rash doesn't spread much beyond the mouth.

Frankly, this was the first and only case of its type I've ever run across in my practice. Nevertheless, I'm including it here because lots of people have been sensitized to poison ivy, and unless they're warned off, many of them are going to eat mangoes.

Do-it-yourself measures won't shorten the episode but should make you feel more comfortable while it lasts—count on at least a week. Self-treatment involves the following:

1. Wash the area with mild soap and water. Rinse thoroughly and blot dry.

2. Apply a clean cloth or sterile gauze pads dipped into salt water (one teaspoon of salt to a pint of very cold water) and wrung out. Hold the compress in place for ten to fifteen minutes.

3. Apply 0.5 percent hydrocortisone cream to affected areas. It should help relieve itching and swelling. Reapply every four hours if necessary.

4. For additional relief, take an over-the-counter oral antihistamine such as Benadryl or Chlor-Trimeton.

Of course, if itching and swelling are severe, see a doctor. He or she might decide to prescribe oral cortisone or administer cortisone by injection in addition to a stronger steroid cream.

Crinkles Around Lips

Many of my patients have told me that they don't mind crinkles at the corners of their eyes, because these lines are associated with laughter. But I've never met anyone who didn't hate the tiny vertical lines radiating from upper and lower lips. Nothing you can buy at a cosmetic counter, or in a drugstore without a prescription, will erase these wrinkles. But there are things you can do to make them less noticeable.

1. Wash your face with mild soap and lukewarm water.
2. Run steaming hot water into bathroom basin or a large, sturdy bowl. Tent a towel over your head and steam your face for about five minutes.
3. While the skin around your mouth is still beaded with steam and perspiration, apply plenty of moisturizer. (Put it on your lips too.) Petroleum jelly is fine for this purpose. So are moisturizers containing collagen or elastin—*not* because these ingredients are absorbed into the skin and strengthen its underlying structure (the molecules are too large to penetrate) but because they help retain moisture.
4. Do the above steps once in the morning, immediately after bath or shower (tissue off excess moisturizer before applying makeup), and once again in the evening, half an hour before bedtime if you have time. "Steam-accelerated" hydration such as this should help plump up skin in the area, making tiny crinkles less noticeable.
5. Once or twice a week, smooth a light oil such as baby oil on your mouth and the skin above your upper lip. Then pick up a small amount of table salt with your oil-moistened index

finger and with very gentle pressure, stroke over the crinkled area on one side of your mouth. *Do not rub salt on your lips. This treatment is for facial skin just above the border of your lips.* Work back and forth from mid-mouth to corner. Pick up more salt and repeat on the other side. Then rinse the area and steam and moisturize as described in steps 2 through 4. Gentle abrasion will slough away old, dead skin cells, exposing younger cells capable of absorbing and retaining more moisture.

IMPORTANT: If your skin is sensitive, use baking soda, a much gentler abrasive than salt. If you skin is *very* sensitive, even baking soda might be too irritating; discontinue treatment if redness and/or soreness result. If you have a cold sore, pimple, or other problem in the area above your lips, wait till it has cleared up before using salt or baking soda.

Blocking Lipstick Bleedthrough

Nothing calls attention to around-the-mouth crinkles like lip-color that has feathered and "bled" into them. Fortunately, many cosmetics companies have taken note of the problem and come up with pre-lipstick bases, or primers, designed to keep color where it belongs. (Elizabeth Arden's Lip-Fix and Max Factor's Lip Renew are two that come to mind.) Use according to instructions that come with the product.

Another way to keep color from straying into tiny lines around your lips is to prep your mouth with foundation. Smooth it on over mouth and lips, stretching the skin very gently so that makeup flows into crinkles. Wait a few minutes to allow foundation to set. Then, with a fresh cotton ball, press loose translucent powder over the entire mouth area. Finally, use a lip pencil or brush to outline your mouth. Fill in with color from the tube.

How to Keep Your Mouth Crinkle-Free Longer

I've seen seventy-year-olds without a hint of wrinkling above their upper lips. I've also seen women in their thirties with noticeable lines in the area. No doubt heredity plays a role in when and whether crinkles appear. But what you do and don't do, starting right now, can also have a major impact.

• Don't smoke. I've mentioned it before, and I'll continue to emphasize the fact that smoking is a first-degree wrinkle promoter. As you puff on a cigarette, muscles around the mouth contract and the overlying skin wrinkles up temporarily. Do it often enough, and temporary wrinkling can become permanent.

• Avoid unnecessary grimacing. Like smoking, habitually puckering or pursing your lips, or distorting them in exaggerated facial gesturing, can hasten the development of lines around the mouth. But don't be afraid to smile a lot. A pleasant expression is the best cosmetic of all.

• Don't neglect your teeth. Those cartoon depictions of toothless old folks with heavy lines on upper and lower lips are based on reality. Teeth are an important part of the underlying support structure of mouth and lips. Without that structure, skin in the mouth area "collapses" and wrinkles. Good dental care—including an immediate implant should you lose a tooth—can help deter premature aging in the area.

• Don't skip sunscreen for your lips and the area immediately surrounding them. Use it every time you go outdoors to protect the area from rays that result in early wrinkling. There's a wide and growing range of sun protection options. For the skin around your mouth, you can use an oil- or water-based product under your makeup. Or you can use a foundation makeup containing sunscreening ingredients. Whichever you choose, of course, key it to your skin type.

You'll need a second, separate product for your lips, since

lip skin is structurally and functionally different from face and body skin. There are literally dozens of different sunscreening lip lubricants and balms from which to select. Or you can wear a lipstick or gloss formulated to block out harmful rays.

For all-day protection, a single morning application is not enough. Though many sunscreens are waterproof, they're not permanent. Touch up after meals and at frequent intervals in between if you are a habitual lip licker or if the weather is hot, causing you to perspire freely.

• Do keep the area surrounding your mouth well moisturized. In speaking with patients, I find that many women—even some who are careful about moisturizing the rest of their face—make a detour around the skin above the upper lip. Even though this area is technically well within the oil-prone "T-zone," it's rarely oily. More often, skin above the mouth needs extra moisture. Don't skip it.

• Don't be overzealous about removing hair above your upper lip. One reason men tend to have fewer wrinkles in the area is because their facial hair, and the follicles from which it grows, is more abundant and supplies additional support to skin. I'm not suggesting that you grow a mustache! But in dealing with upper lip fuzz, keep in mind that electrolysis, which destroys the follicles, and waxing, which pulls hair out by the roots, decrease the amount of underlying skin support. From a wrinkle-deterring perspective, a depilatory, which dissolves hair at or slightly below the skin surface, is a better choice. If the growth above your upper lip is fine and sparse, bleaching, which leaves hairs intact, might be better still.

Permanent Solutions

Upper-lip crinkling doesn't have to be forever. In some instances, Retin-A, applied nightly or every other night for a period of months, renders them less visible. Chemical peeling or dermabrasion will erase fine to medium lines. Collagen injections can fill in deeper ones. Of course, these wrinkle-fixing techniques must be supervised or performed by a dermatologist. For more about these procedures, see Chapter 9.

Blue Lipstick

There's probably nothing wrong with you or your lipstick if it turns slightly bluish soon after you apply it. Individual skin chemistry varies and can affect certain lipstick formulations in different ways—usually by shifting true reds and even corals over toward the purplish end of the color spectrum. You can't do anything to modify your skin chemistry, but there are ways to prevent unflattering changes in the color of your lipstick.

• "Block" the chemical interactions that cause "blueing." Before applying lipstick, smooth foundation over your mouth. Allow it to dry. Dust on loose, transparent or "no-color" powder. Stroke lipstick on over powder. The two cosmetics—foundation and powder—should be enough to run interference between skin and lip color, allowing the latter to remain true.
• Counteract the shift to blue with a gold-toned lip primer. (These products are also sometimes called lip bases, lip foundations, and lipstick undercoats.) Apply liberally and blot. Finish with lipstick. If one coat of primer doesn't prevent lip color from turning bluish, try two, blotting after each one.
• To get an idea of whether and how much a lipstick color will change on your lips, give it a trial run before buying. Stroke a small amount from the store tester tube on the inside of your wrist and wait ten minutes. (If you're considering a lip color for day wear, go outside, where the store lighting won't interfere with it, to make a final judgment.)
• Keep in mind that frosted formulations and sheer, glossy products on lips tend to change less than creamy lipsticks.

Choosing Lip Colors That Flatter

To judge how well a color harmonizes with your skin tone, eyes, and hair, stroke tester color on your wrist and wait ten minutes. Then hold your wrist up to your face and study the effect in a mirror. Smile as you do so. If your teeth have a dark or yellowish cast, watch out for lipsticks in the orange family. They'll emphasize the yellow. Likewise, if your teeth are a grayish or bluish shade, burgundy, plum, and other lipsticks with a bluish undertone will make your teeth seem dingier.

Dark or brilliant reds, bright oranges, and intense pinks call attention to the lower half of your face. That's good if your mouth is your best feature, if the skin around it is clear, firm, and relatively unlined, and if your teeth are even and white. Otherwise, choose softer, subtler shades.

5

Help for Hair

One of the things I try to make clear to patients is that while there isn't a "cure" for every hair problem, *something* can almost always be done to make their hair look and behave better—sometimes a lot better. In this chapter I'll tell you about the products and procedures that will help you deal with thinning hair, fine or skimpy hair, dryness, oiliness, breakage, and other common problems. Let's start with the most distressing problem, hair that seems to be getting thinner.

Thinning Hair

Thinning hair is alarming to anyone—whether male or female. Though thinning can be a "normal" consequence of natural changes in hormone production, it can also be due to poor health, a side effect of certain kinds of medication, or the result of mistreatment. Let's look in more detail at the causes of hair loss and what can be done about the problem.

The Whys of Thinning Hair

If you've been pregnant, you may have noticed that your hair gradually became thicker and softer as the pregnancy progressed. That was because your body was producing more estrogen. But after childbirth, when estrogen levels tapered off, hair growth may have slowed and you might have been upset by increased fallout. Many cases of thinning hair can be traced to a decrease in estrogen, the female hormone that plays such an important role in reproduction. Fortunately, postpartum thinning is usually temporary; hair almost always returns to its prepregnancy state within months. However, a dermatologist can speed things along by prescribing topical preparations containing estrogen, progesterone, or steroids, or by injecting cortisone into the scalp.

Birth control pills are sometimes a factor in hair loss. Those containing the synthetic male hormone androgen can increase fallout. (Androgen, not so coincidentally, is also a factor in male thinning and baldness.) Oral contraceptives made with estrogen, on the other hand, often make hair thicker and more lustrous, but when they are discontinued there may be significant thinning, which may not be noticeable until two or three months later. The important thing is not to panic. Loss of hair related to the use of birth control pills of either kind almost always corrects itself within months after pill use is stopped.

Stress, which can trigger production of larger than usual amounts of male hormones in women, sometimes has the same effect as taking birth control pills containing androgen: increased hair fallout. A single psychological trauma or ongoing tension can do it. In fact, I believe—as do many of my colleagues—that the recent rise in female baldness has a lot to do with the greater stress associated with the conflicting demands of job, home, and child-rearing.

Stress-related thinning can occur at any age and may or may not reverse itself without medical intervention. But help is available if you need it. Among the treatments your dermatologist might decide to use are lotions containing estrogen or progesterone, progesterone drops or injections, topically applied or injected steroids, and oral thyroid preparations.

Diminished estrogen production during menopause is another hormone-related cause of hair loss. (The diameter of the hair shaft sometimes "shrinks" with age, adding to the problem.) Without medical intervention, hair fallout related to menopause is permanent. The drug Rogaine may help, however, and for some women, hair transplants work well. (More about Rogaine and transplants later in this chapter.)

In some women, certain over-the-counter and prescription drugs can result in hair loss as an unwanted side effect. The most commonly used of these drugs are:

Accutane, used for treating acne
anti-ulcer drugs
aspirin (in large doses, over long periods)
boric acid, an ingredient in some mouthwashes
cholesterol-lowering agents
a few prescription arthritis medications
iodides in cough medicines
some antidepressants

If thinning is a consequence of taking medicine, the problem usually goes away when the drugs are discontinued.

Diet can also affect hair. Too much wheat germ, for example, seems to promote male hormone production—and hair fallout—in women. Overdosing on vitamins A and E, and the minerals iodine and selenium, can have a negative effect. The same is true of crash dieting. Because of protein deprivation, some strict vegetarians experience hair loss. (Hair, literally made of protein, needs a plentiful dietary supply of this nutrient for its formation and growth.) Iron deficiency, caused by an iron-poor diet (or occasionally by very heavy menstrual flow), can also result in thinning. In fact, any great deviation from normal nutrition for any length of time will result in temporary hair loss that may take two or three months to become apparent. In those cases where inadequate nutrition has resulted in hair loss, a return to a well-balanced diet is the most effective "medicine," though in some instances a dermatologist will prescribe hormone lotions, drops, or injections to accelerate new hair growth.

Poor health and certain illnesses sometimes lead to thinning. A high fever, whatever the cause, can result in noticeable fallout weeks or months later. Thyroid abnormalities, liver or kidney dysfunction, and the trauma of surgery are also potential causes of hair loss. Once again, the condition usually improves without medical intervention when physical well-being is restored. If progress is slow, a dermatologist may be able to stimulate quicker regrowth.

One thing many of my patients are unaware of is the fact that thinning is a possible side effect of cosmetic plastic surgery. It can be an unpleasant, even frightening, surprise if the patient has not been informed. I have no doubt that most surgeons tell their patients ahead of time about the possible complications and side effects of the surgery to be performed, but some apparently neglect to mention hair loss. Several times I've had people come into my office in a state of near-hysteria because of mysterious thinning occurring soon after plastic surgery. One woman, whose hair was skimpy to begin with, had a combination face lift and brow lift (a procedure in which forehead lines are smoothed by removing excess skin from along an incision across the top of the head behind the hairline). A few weeks after the operation, when she got the okay from her surgeon to resume normal shampooing and styling, she was horrified to see how much *less* hair she had to work with. We had one of those good news/bad news talks. I told her that thinning due to the shock of surgery would most probably reverse itself in time. But hair lost along the scar resulting from the incision was gone for good.

Another cause of hair loss can be a bad case of dandruff (*seborrheic dermatitis*), characterized by patches of severe scaling and redness. An anti-dandruff regimen and, if necessary, topical or oral medication prescribed by a dermatologist, should clear up the condition and set the stage for new hair growth.

Then there is thinning caused by abuse. Chemical overprocessing—careless or too-frequent perming, coloring, straightening, etc.—can make hair so brittle and weak, even gentle combing and brushing results in breakage and fallout. I'm tempted to call this "do-it-yourselfer's syndrome" because most cases of severe chemical damage I've seen are self-inflicted. A woman will give herself a perm, and if she doesn't like the results, she'll reperm just a few days later. Or she'll lighten her hair and then, dissatisfied with the color, run out and buy a permanent dye to correct it. Or she'll perm and color in the same week. I have nothing against home perms and home hair-coloring kits. Used exactly according to manufacturers' instructions, they're no harder on hair than the more costly salon procedures and often produce results that are every bit as good. It's *overuse* that gets people into trouble. Still, the hair follicle is not affected by overprocessing, so if hair is given a long vacation from chemical processing, new growth should be normal and as thick as ever. (I *do* advise, however, that home hair-straightening kits be avoided. Chemical straighteners are harsher than home perming, waving, and coloring products, and if I had my way, my patients would never use them.)

Rough handling sometimes leads to what is called *traction alopecia*, in which hair is broken or torn out when it is pulled tight and set on rollers, braided, or done in a tight ponytail or chignon. (Among my hair-loss patients have been several preteens, brought in by their worried mothers. In each case the daughter was a serious ballet student who pulled her hair into a bun for class each day.) Even overvigorous brushing, combing, and teasing can pull out enough hair to result in noticeable thinning. Traction alopecia is rarely permanent. Unless follicles are damaged, new hair sprouts and grows on schedule. In the meantime, it's important to treat hair more gently.

So far I've been discussing *alopecia areata*—thinning linked to hormone changes, stress, illness, or physical trauma. There is another kind of hair loss, which is genetically "programmed." This is characterized by diffuse thinning across the entire top of the scalp and, sometimes, a receding hairline. (The pattern is similar to that seen in men, but in women progresses much more slowly and almost never leads to total balding.) A family history of significant hair loss—among male *and* female relatives—is one tip-off that thinning is hereditary. Genetic hair loss can begin in early adulthood; I've treated many women in their thirties, and even a few in their twenties, who were losing hair at the crown. Unfortunately, this kind of thinning doesn't reverse itself, nor does it respond to any medication you can buy without a prescription. But, as I'll explain in the treatment section that follows, the situation isn't hopeless.

Rx for Hair Loss

Not long ago, the only way to deal with certain kinds of hair loss was to invest in a good wig. In some cases a well-made, attractively styled wig is still the only beauty solution. But more and more types of thinning and balding can be treated today, thanks to advances in medical science.

In stubborn cases of alopecia areata, dermatologists sometimes obtain strikingly good results by injecting cortisone directly into the problem area. When it works, new growth tends to be lighter in color and finer in texture, but in time begins to resemble more closely hair on other parts of the head. As I've mentioned, treatments include topically applied steroids, topical anthralin creams, and oral thyroid extracts, if appropriate. If one course of treatment fails, a second or third procedure often will be successful.

For genetic hair loss, characterized by top-of-the-head thinning, minoxidil, approved by the FDA for treating hair loss in 1988, and now marketed under the name Rogaine, can be the answer. This topically administered preparation isn't an overnight problem-solver. New hair growth, if it occurs, may not be evident until several months after treatment has begun. And to maintain good results, drug applications must be continued on a regular basis thereafter. As for the chances of success with minoxidil/Rogaine, studies conducted by Upjohn, the manufacturer, indicated that the drug grows cosmetically acceptable hair in about 30 percent of patients. (When used in conjunction with Retin-A, Rogaine appears to be somewhat more effective.) But even when it doesn't actually cause new hair to sprout, this remarkable drug often halts further thinning.

The ideal candidate for treatment with Rogaine is under forty, someone who began to lose hair fairly recently, and whose bald spots, if any, are relatively small. Interestingly, the drug often works better for women than for men. Rogaine can be effective in cases of "genetic" hair loss and occasionally for *alopecia areata*; it doesn't help when balding is a result of disease, thyroid hormone deficiency, or skin disorders. And it won't grow hair where there is total baldness. Rogaine is not a miracle drug after all, but it has helped many men and women look better and feel better about themselves. If you want to explore this option, see a dermatologist who has a special interest in the problem of hair loss and who is experienced in the use of minoxidil/Rogaine.

Hair transplants are another possible solution to thinning or balding—assuming, of course, that there is enough good, healthy hair on the scalp to be uprooted and relocated. The procedure is performed in a dermatologist's office under local anesthesia. Fifty or more tiny sections, or plugs, each containing a few hairs, are cut and lifted from donor areas of the scalp. An equal number of tiny notches are cut into the bald area. The plugs are trimmed and fitted snugly into the notches. Typically, hair in the donor plugs falls out and follicles lie dormant for about three months after the shock of relocation. When new hair makes its appearance, it is often curlier and not as dense as hair in the area from which it was taken, but rapidly assumes the characteristics of donor areas.

Depending on the size of the area to be filled in, one or more additional sessions may be necessary. At a cost of $25 and up per plug, transplants aren't cheap. But for those who agonize over hair loss, results can be worth it.

Is hair transplantation for you? The only way to know for sure is to consult a dermatologist. Major considerations are the extent of hair loss, hair type (curly, coarse, dark hair fills in better than fine, light hair), and medical history. People with high blood pressure, bleeding disorders, and a tendency to scar badly are poor candidates. However, age alone is rarely a problem. I've performed successful hair transplantation on women who are well into their sixties.

Some other surgical options are worth mentioning. In flap surgery, a long, narrow C-shaped section of hair-bearing scalp is removed and relocated to the bald area on top of the head.

The advantage is that large amounts of hair can be transplanted all at once. The procedure is a more drastic operation than ordinary hair transplantation and not for everyone.

Scalp reduction surgery is another possibility, but only if your scalp is healthy and elastic. Here, a narrow section of scalp is removed from the balding area. Then the two edges are pulled together and sutured closed, decreasing the size of the bald patch. Surgery may need to be repeated several times to eliminate the bald area.

What Not to Do About Thinning Hair

Hair loss can be extremely distressing, especially to a woman. Distress fosters vulnerability. The person with thinning hair may be so desperate to reverse or at least halt the hair loss process, he or she will try *any* pill, potion, or procedure—no matter how outlandish or potentially harmful—that promises results.

The treatments I've touched on in this chapter have been used successfully, though they do not work equally well for everyone. Unfortunately, I can't say the same about megadoses of vitamins, scalp manipulation, and the vast array of over-the-counter baldness "cures" advertised in newspapers, magazines, and elsewhere. If any of them were truly effective, *everyone* would know about it, and no one would agonize anymore about hair loss. A certain amount of skepticism can save you money and aggravation.

I also urge you to be wary of certain procedures that *do* work but are loaded with drawbacks and risks. In hair weaving, for example, your own hair is used to anchor a hairpiece to your scalp. The process can damage existing hair and must be repeated as it grows—otherwise the hairpiece will loosen and lift off. In another procedure, hair implantation, a hairpiece is sutured to the scalp. Ongoing soreness in the sutured area is not uncommon, and there is a possibility of scarring, which can destroy healthy hair follicles. Another drawback is that brushing, combing, shampooing, et cetera, tend to pull individual hairs from the hairpiece.

When thinning is a problem, the very best advice I can give is: See a dermatologist and get the facts as they pertain to *you*. Don't proceed with treatment until these key questions have been answered to your satisfaction: Are you a good candidate for the proposed technique? What is the risk to the hair you have left and to your overall well-being and comfort? What is the likelihood of satisfactory results?

Note that hair can *seem* thin because it's fine or because of an insufficiency of follicles. These factors are genetically deter-mined. There's nothing "wrong" with your hair if it's skimpy for either reason. The following section tells you how to make fine or skimpy hair appear thicker.

Fine or Skimpy Hair

I know a few people who think their hair is too thick, but they're a small minority. A far more common complaint is not enough hair. I sometimes hear it from patients who actually have plenty of hair. But because it's baby fine or lacks body, it seems skimpier than it is. Other people really do have skimpy hair. Either way, though, it's possible to get the look of more hair.

How to Get "Fatter" Hair in Less Than Four Hours

Use a shampoo and conditioner formulated to add body. These can be identified by the words "body building" or "extra body" on the label. Check the ingredient listing to make sure it con-tains one or more of the following: proteins (keratin and col-lagen are proteins), silicone polymers, polymeric quaternium compounds. These substances cling to the hair shaft, making it seem thicker.

Use styling aids such as mousse, gel, setting lotion, and spray to add fullness. After shampooing and towel drying, place a small amount in the palm of one hand. Rub your hands together to distribute the product. Weave fingers through your hair and apply the product to roots only. Don't massage it in. Instead, lift and "scrunch" hair at the scalp, especially at the crown, back, and in other areas where you want more fullness. Allow your hair to air dry. If time is short, use a blow-dryer fitted with a diffuser (these devices are available in the hair appliance sections of well-stocked department and specialty stores). With a diffuser, the rush of air from a dryer is tamed so that lift and volume aren't blown out.

If hair goes flat during the day, reactivate the styling product you used earlier by wetting your hands, shaking off excess moisture, and repeating the lifting/scrunching maneuvers described above.

Back-comb it. Gentle teasing with a comb or brush will build in more height and volume. Done properly, it won't hurt your hair: Lift a small section of hair in one hand. With comb or brush held in the other hand, *lightly* stroke hair toward scalp. Three or four strokes per section should be enough to add fullness. Finish by blending other hair over back-combed sections.

Color it. The chemicals in many hair-color products lift and roughen the *cuticle* (the cells that make up the outermost layer of the hair shaft), increasing its diameter and making it seem thicker. If your hair is "virgin"—not previously colored, permed, or straightened—and in good condition, brightening, lightening, or intensifying its natural color could give you the look and feel of more abundant tresses. Only products designated as "permanent" or "semi-permanent" will achieve these results, however. Temporary color, the kind that lasts through just a few shampoos, merely coats hair with a semi-transparent film.

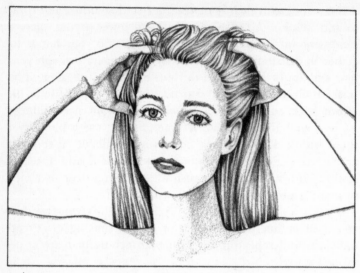

A

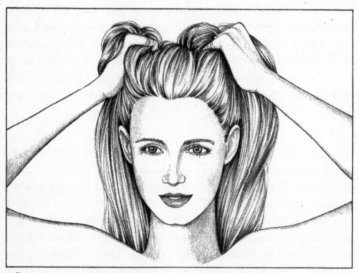

B

To give hair more volume, place a small amount of styling gel, setting lotion, or mousse in the palms of your hands. Weave fingers through hair (A), then "scrunch" close to the scalp (B).

Get a perm. Even when it's skimpy, a head of curly or wavy hair tends to look thicker than it is because it takes up more space than straight hair. And, like semi-permanent and permanent hair color, permanent wave solutions fatten individual hairs by roughing up the cuticle. (Some salons will apply perm solutions without rolling the hair in rods to give hair bulk without curl.) Perming is not a good idea, though, when hair is in poor condition, because chemicals used in the process can further weaken fragile, damaged locks.

Change the style. Straight hair seems to have more volume when it's blunt cut so that individual hairs stack up, one on top of the other. Curly or wavy hair looks thicker cut in layers. As a general rule, short to medium-length hair seems fuller than long hair, which tends to be flattened and dragged down by its own weight. And long hair, unless it is frequently trimmed, is often sparse and scraggly at the ends because of splits, uneven growth, and breakage farther up the shaft.

Damaged Hair

I seem to see more and more dull, dry, brittle hair in my practice these days. In most cases it's not hard to discover the cause: improper or too-frequent perming, straightening, or coloring, careless use of dryers, heated curlers, and other appliances. The awful truth is hair that has been tortured by chemicals or subjected to physical abuse is beyond repair. Damage to the hair shaft is permanent. Hurt hair won't return to "normal" until the damaged portions have grown out and been cut off. However, it is possible to improve the look, feel, and manageability of abused locks.

Two-Step Crash Plan for Sick Hair

1. Have your hair trimmed or, better still, cut. The tip ends of hair are oldest and have taken the most abuse; newer hair,

closer to the scalp, is always in better condition. Snipping off several inches eliminates much of the problem. After your initial cut or trim, have hair shaped every four to six weeks. Succeeding trims should bring tangible improvement as the proportion of hurt hair to healthy is altered in favor of the latter.

2. Give hair a deep conditioning treatment. You can have this done at a salon, as a follow-up to a cut or trim, or you can do it yourself. Either way, make sure that the conditioning product contains large amounts of a protein ingredient, such as hydrolyzed animal protein, collagen, or keratin. (Protein adheres to the hair shaft, filling in cracks and breaks, almost like plaster, making hair temporarily smoother and stronger.) For deepest conditioning, the product should be applied with heat and left on the hair for fifteen to thirty minutes.

To get the benefits of heat, use a dryer with a plastic bonnet. If you don't have one, apply conditioner, pile hair on top of your head, and wrap with clear plastic wrap. Wrap again with a towel or other cloth wrung out of very warm water. When the towel begins to cool, dunk it in more warm water, wring, and rewrap. Repeat for fifteen to thirty minutes.

Treat damaged hair to deep conditioning at least once a week.

A Regimen for Dry, Damaged Hair

Chemical processing, careless use of heat-generating appliances, rough handling, and exposure to environmental extremes all tend to lift and roughen the cuticle—the cells that make up the outer layer of the hair shaft. Roughened cuticle doesn't reflect light as well as smooth, normal cuticle, which is why dry or damaged hair often looks dull. With further abuse, portions of the cuticle can be worn away, causing hair to become strawlike and brittle. (Severely abused hair may feel "gummy" when wet.)

Though lost cuticle can't be restored, proteinized intensive conditioners can help smooth it. However, nothing that comes in a jar or bottle will do as much for dry, damaged hair as gentle treatment. The following dos and don'ts should prove helpful.

• Do shampoo only as often as necesssary to keep hair clean. With the advent of wash-and-wear styles, daily shampooing has become the norm for many women. There's nothing wrong with that if hair is in good condition. However, I tell my patients with damaged hair to wait at least three or four days between shampoos to minimize exposure to alkaline ingredients that strip away oil and can cause additional erosion of the cuticle.

Some of my patients insist that their hair is easier to manage after a shampoo. However, manageability is probably not the result of using a cleansing product, but of thoroughly wetting—"moisturizing"—the hair with water. If you too believe your hair behaves better, and feels softer and more flexible, after a shampoo, see if you don't get the same results from simply rinsing your hair in plain water and following up with an instant conditioner made for dry, permed, or color-treated hair. Do this every day if you like and save "real" shampooing for once or twice a week.

The best shampoos for hurt hair are those labeled for dry, permed, color-treated, or damaged hair. Use the product sparingly—about half as much as the amount suggested on the label is enough. Dampen hair first with warm, not hot, water, then concentrate lather on scalp and the hair closest to it. Instead of rubbing suds into fragile ends, squeeze through briefly. Work quickly. Do not allow suds to remain any longer than it takes to get hair clean. Do not relather. Rinse thoroughly with warm water.

• Do follow each shampoo or rinsing with an instant conditioner that makes combing easier and encourages the cuticle to lie flatter. Almost every major hair care company makes an instant conditioner labeled for damaged, dry, permed, or color-treated hair. Some of the best contain quaternium compounds (often designated by a number, such as 23, in the ingredient list) and hydrolyzed animal protein, keratin, or collagen. Not all of these products are meant to be rinsed out. Some work best when left on the hair. Check labels to determine which kind you are buying.

When you are making your selection, you may notice some conditioners that feature a pH factor of 6, 5, 4, or even 3 on the label. The lower the pH factor, the more acidic the product and the better it is for damaged hair. Low pH formulas tend to have a smoothing effect on the cuticle and help to make hair shinier, less porous, and easier to comb.

• Do detangle wet hair gently and carefully. Use a good comb with smoothly rounded, widely spaced teeth. Work on a small section at a time. Start an inch or so from the ends, combing gently down to the tips. If you hit a snarl, try to undo most of it with your fingers. When the ends of a section are tangle-free, move up to hair closer to the scalp. Hair is weakest when wet, so *never* yank through damp hair with a comb, and don't even think about brushing it till it's dry.

• Do allow damaged hair to dry naturally, whenever possible, since hot air from a blow-dryer can do additional damage to the cuticle. When you can't wait for hair to dry on its own, blot up as much moisture as possible with a towel. Then use a dryer on the low, or cool, setting. Keep the dryer at least nine inches away from your hair, and don't focus the flow of air on one area for more than a few seconds.

• Don't use a curling iron, electric rollers, or other heat-producing stylers until your hair is in better shape; heat from these appliances can further roughen and erode the cuticle. (Some of the worst cases of hair damage I've seen were due to improper use of these tools.) On special occasions, when you *must* use one of these stylers, apply to hair as briefly as possible and set the temperature control at low.

• Don't use hairpins, barrettes, clips, rubber bands, et cetera, since these, too, can break weak, brittle hair.

• Do protect your hair from weather extremes by tucking it up under a hat or covering it with a scarf. Raw winter wind and hot summer sun can be almost as hard on hair as they are on skin.

• Don't brush your hair 100 strokes a day. If your hair is very weak and brittle, don't brush it at all, since bristles pulled through damaged hair can break it or pull it out. To get more blood flowing to your scalp and duplicate the pleasant, tingling sensation that is a side benefit of brushing, lean over and massage your scalp gently for a few minutes with your fingers.

• Don't perm, straighten, or color your hair. If it's already permed or colored, this guideline may be the hardest of all to follow since the growing-out stage is always awkward. Nevertheless, resist the temptation to reperm or recolor damaged hair; further chemical processing will cancel out anything else you do to help it back to health.

Dry Hair

All badly damaged hair is dry, but not all dry hair is badly damaged. It may be "naturally" dry in the sense that oil glands in the scalp are underactive. Or it may be that a dry climate or indoor environment, overexposure to sun and wind, over-vigorous cleansing, overprocessing, or overuse of hair appliances has removed enough moisture from the hair shaft to make locks look dull and feel harsh instead of shiny and soft. Nevertheless, if your hair is dry, it will benefit from the care guidelines given earlier for damaged hair.

You can also try the following do-it-yourself treatments. Use them when you run out of your favorite commercial conditioner or any time your hair needs a change of pace.

Mayonnaise Deep Conditioner for Dry Hair

Look at the ingredient list on a jar of mayonnaise, and you'll see that it contains substances similar to those in many commercial conditioners: protein (in this case eggs), an acid (vinegar), and lots of oil.

1. Measure out about one-quarter cup of mayonnaise.

2. Wet your hair thoroughly with warm water, blot up excess, then apply mayonnaise, paying special attention to the ends.

3. Wrap your hair turban-style in a towel wrung out of warm water, or cover your hair with clear plastic wrap.

4. Wait fifteen to thirty minutes, then shampoo and rinse thoroughly.

Egg and Yogurt Dry Hair Conditioner

This one takes a few tablespoons of plain yogurt and an egg. Mix thoroughly in a cup or small bowl, then apply as above.

How to Refresh Dry Hair in Seven Minutes

In the middle of the day, or anytime dry hair becomes flyaway and out of control, the following treatment will help calm it down and revitalize the style. It's good for permed and naturally curly hair, as well as straight hair. Don't use it if you set your hair on rollers, since the moisture involved will loosen curls and waves.

You'll need a small amount of cream rinse, or instant conditioner and water. If you're away from home and have neither with you, you could use hand lotion. You will also need hairspray.

1. Dampen your hands with water. Pour a few drops of cream rinse, conditioner, or hand lotion into your palms, then "comb" through your hair with your fingers. The idea is *not* to wet your hair, but to deliver the moisture it needs to make it behave.

2. Repeat if necessary, patting more water and cream rinse on areas that are most out of control, such as the ends and the hair around your face.

3. Wait a couple of minutes, then finger-comb your hair into place. Finish with hairspray to keep it in line.

Oily Hair

You don't need an expert to diagnose oily hair. If it begins to feel and look greasy and if strands begin to separate and clump together soon after shampooing—sometimes within just a few hours—it's oily.

The almost-instant oil-blotting treatment that follows can save the day when you're rushing to a meeting or social engagement and there's no time to wash your hair.

Five-Minute Emergency De-greaser

Dry shampoo works best, but almost any absorbent powdery substance—such as face or baby powder, talc, cornstarch, even baking powder—can be substituted. You'll also need some hair-spray.

1. Since oil is probably concentrated at your hairline in front, and along your part if you wear one, sprinkle a small amount of dry shampoo or powder into the palms of your hands and work it into those areas only.
2. Brush your hair to remove as much shampoo or powder as possible.
3. Control static flyaways (a consequence of this oil-removal technique) and remove remaining traces of shampoo or powder by running a brush sprayed with hairspray through your hair.

Basics of Oily Hair Care

The most important thing you can do for oily hair is to keep it clean without overmanipulating your scalp. Stimulating the scalp tends to cause an increase in oil output.

I recommend daily shampooing to my patients with oily hair. Products labeled for oily hair are best. These usually contain one or more of the following aggressive cleansers: ammonium lauryl sulfate, sodium lauryl sulfate, sodium olefin sulfate. Avoid "moisturizing" and "conditioning" shampoos and rinses which may not have the cleaning power you need, and which are made with oily ingredients that can aggravate your problem.

To shampoo oily hair, dampen it first, then lather up. Massage suds gently and briefly onto scalp and squeeze through hair ends. Rinse thoroughly with cool water (hot and even warm water can stimulate oil gland activity). Finish with conditioner made for oily hair. Or try a simple do-it-yourself lemon or vinegar rinse:

Add two tablespoons vinegar (white vinegar if your hair is light) or one teaspoon lemon juice to one and one-half quarts cool water and mix. Pour through hair, squeeze through strands for thirty seconds. Then rinse thoroughly with cold water.

Many of my patients have "combination" hair—oily at the scalp but dry at the ends. If this is your problem, try the preceding method of shampooing, but use a product for normal hair. You can follow up with "combination" conditioning. The method that follows helps moisturize dry ends without adding oily ingredients to an already too-oily scalp.

Post-Shampoo Conditioning for Half-and-Half Hair

1. Pour a small amount of cream rinse or conditioner made for dry hair into a cup or small container.
2. Add water and swirl to mix.
3. Dunk hair ends *only* into rinse or conditioner. Wait two or three minutes. Then rinse thoroughly.

• If your scalp is very oily, you might want to try de-greasing every few days with an astringent lotion (it could be the same one you use on your face) or witch hazel: After shampooing, part your hair, dip a cotton ball in astringent, squeeze out excess, then dab along the part. Continue parting and dabbing until you've treated your entire scalp.

• Don't use any oil-based product on oily hair. If it needs help holding a style, use products with an alcohol or water base. Do

not massage styling products into roots. Instead, apply them
starting two or three inches from your scalp.

• Assuming the ends of your hair are not overly dry, a body
wave or perm might be a good idea since the chemicals in these
products have a drying effect and can make hair look and feel
less limp and greasy. The same is true of permanent hair-color
products (those that do not wash out). Incidentally, it's not necessary to make a drastic change in the color of your hair to get
these benefits; you could choose a shade that matches or is very
close to your own.

After you perm or color, reassess the condition of your hair.
Processing could dry it enough to require changes in the way
you care for it. Depending on the degree of dryness, for example, you might need to shampoo less often, or use milder
products, perhaps made for normal hair or even dry hair.

Commonsense Advice for Every Hair Type

• Protect your hair from the sun. There are dozens of hair
products containing sunscreening ingredients, and some of
them can be helpful in minimizing sun damage. But in my
opinion, none of them are as effective as wearing a scarf or
hat. My patients frequently protest. "It's too hot at the beach
for a scarf." Well, maybe. Polyester and other synthetic fabrics
that do not "breathe" can be uncomfortably warm. But that's
not the case with cotton or silk, or with a loosely woven straw
hat, which allow cooling air to circulate through the weave.

Keep in mind that blond hair, like fair skin, tends to be more
vulnerable to sun damage. The same goes for hair that is dry,
permed, or color-treated. (When it is well protected from the
sun, chemically lightened hair is less subject to oxidation, the
process that turns the color orangy, or "brassy.")

• Protect your hair from chlorinated pool water and salt water,
two more potential hair hazards that can dry and damage the

cuticle. (Once again, fragile dry and/or chemically treated hair is especially susceptible.) And chlorine can give bleached and natural blond hair a peculiar greenish or bluish cast. Take precautions: Wear a bathing cap for swimming. For extra protection, apply a few drops of cream rinse or a light oil, such as baby oil, to your hair, then pile hair on top of your head and pull on a cap. Some dedicated swimmers further "waterproof" their hair by wrapping a length of chamois around it before putting on a bathing cap.

After swimming, shampoo or rinse your hair thoroughly in clear water.

I once got a frantic call from a patient who didn't wear a cap when she went swimming at a local pool. Her hair had turned an awful green, she said, and shampooing hadn't helped. Did I have any suggestions for getting the green out? Frankly, I was stumped and had to do some research. I came up with the following:

A teaspoon of citric acid (available at pharmacies) mixed in one-half quart lukewarm water and poured several times through hair sometimes neutralizes swimming pool green. Finish by shampooing and conditioning as usual.

Or wash your hair with one of the special shampoos formulated to undo the effects of chlorine. UltraSwim is one. Use it according to directions on the label.

Or try one of the new "deep cleaning" shampoos, formulated to remove product buildup. Redken Hair Cleansing Creme, for example, is marketed as a good choice for lifting various substances from the hair shaft, including chlorine green.

• Inspect hair tools from time to time and get rid of anything that can snag or break hair—such as bobby pins that have lost their protective plastic tips, combs with broken or missing teeth, metal clips with sharp or rough edges. Do not use plain rubber bands to secure a ponytail or chignon; they can't be removed without also pulling out several strands of hair. Much better are those elastic-coated bands made especially to hold hair in place.

• Brush your hair just enough to keep it looking fresh and groomed and to remove surface dirt. Remember, too much brushing can result in breakage if hair is damaged and can make oily hair oilier. *Never* brush your hair when it's wet, or when it is heavily coated with hairspray, mousse, or other styling product.

I'm often asked what kind of brush is best. Actually, it depends on your hair. Bristles should be soft enough not to scratch your scalp, and long enough and strong enough to penetrate several layers of hair. Thus a brush with soft, short, natural bristles is best for fine hair that is not especially thick. Longer, somewhat stiffer bristles may be needed to get through thick fine hair or hair that is medium in texture. For coarse, thick, or wiry hair, only the longest, stiffest bristles will do the job. Natural bristles tend to be easiest on the hair, but don't be satisfied with just any natural brush. Before buying a brush, natural or synthetic, check to make sure the bristles are smooth enough not to snag hair.

• Sometimes hair benefits from a switch in products. (It's almost as if it gets bored with the same old shampoo and conditioner and welcomes a change of pace.) For example, a brand that helped make your hair shiny and manageable for months might, gradually or suddenly, leave it dull and limp. When something like this happens, it's a signal to reassess your hair and consider changing to another type of product or products (if the condition of your hair has changed) or simply try a different manufacturer's version of the same product. Either way, a variation in your hair care routine could give your hair new life.

Another possibility, when hair suddenly stops behaving as it usually does, is to use one of the relatively new shampoos marketed as "deep cleaning" products. They're formulated to remove buildup deposited by styling aids such as gel, mousse, spray, and so on. A few of my patients who are heavy users of gel and mousse tell me their hair seemed to improve after they shampooed with one of the deep cleaners. (Some of these products apparently clean so well they're too aggressive for regular use and are not recommended for daily shampooing over long periods. If you buy one, be sure to check the label to find out what the manufacturer has to say about how often and how long the product can be used.)

If changing products doesn't revive your hair, ask yourself if you're doing too much—or too little—to it. Overshampooing, for example, can make normal hair feel harsh, almost "crisp," instead of soft and flexible. Washing less often might restore its former texture. On the other hand, when hair that is usually bouncy begins to feel limp or heavy, the solution could be to shampoo more frequently. Adjusting the amount and frequency of conditioning products could also make a difference.

The point I want to make here is that hair and its response to various products can change over time. Normal hair goes through dry periods and oily phases, depending on physical and emotional factors, the season, the environment, and of course on how it's treated. Oily hair can become more or less oily; dry hair can go from slightly dry to very dry. If you're sensitive to these changes and make adjustments in the way you care for it, chances are your hair will look and behave better than if you cling to a single fixed routine.

Dandruff

It's estimated that about 50 percent of the population experiences some flaking of the scalp. Probably because flaky skin is associated with lack of moisture, there's a persistent belief even among many hairdressers and other hair experts that dandruff is a result of excessive dryness. In fact, some of the worst cases I've seen were aggravated by measures intended to combat dryness: greasy pomades, hot olive oil treatments, infrequent shampooing, to name a few.

So-called *ordinary dandruff* flakes are composed of dead skin cells clumped with scalp oils. Another condition, *cosmetic dandruff*, is part dead skin cells and oil, part residue from hairstyling products. Oiling the hair and scalp or failing to remove excess oil through frequent shampooing will compound either type of dandruff.

There's a third and more serious form of dandruff, called

seborrheic dermatitis, characterized by severe flaking, scaling, and even inflammation. It can involve forehead, mid-face, sides of the nose and chin (the T-zone), eyebrows, eyelids, and behind and inside the ears, and in men, the chest. The exact cause of this condition is still unknown, though it's believed that abnormally accelerated cell growth plays a role.

Severe flaking with redness or soreness should be seen by a dermatologist. It could be seborrheic dermatitis, which if untreated, can result in scarring and hair loss. Mild or moderate flaking without redness is probably nothing to worry about, though it can certainly be a source of embarrassment.

How to Get Dandruff Under Control in Fifteen Minutes

When the problem is ordinary or cosmetic dandruff, you should see significant improvement after washing your hair with an over-the-counter antidandruff shampoo containing zinc pirithione (Head & Shoulders, Zincon) or selenium sulfide (Selsun Blue) or sulfur and salicylic acid (Sebulex). These products are formulated to slow the rapid cell turnover associated with the condition. I tell my patients to use these products as follows:

1. Wet your hair thoroughly with lukewarm water, pour a small amount of shampoo into the palm of one hand, then massage onto your scalp. Rinse.
2. Apply more shampoo, massage lather gently onto scalp, and allow it to remain for five minutes.
3. Rinse very thoroughly; loosened flakes will be rinsed out along with the shampoo.
4. Blot up excess moisture with a towel, then allow hair to air dry. If you're in a rush and must use a dryer, switch it to the cool setting and hold it at least six inches from your scalp.

Ordinarily, I recommend daily shampooing with an antidandruff product. To keep the problem under control, it's often necessary to use an antidandruff shampoo on a regular, long-term basis. If that turns out to be the case for you, be sure to change to a different product every three or four weeks. These shampoos tend to lose their effectiveness with prolonged use owing to the development of an immunity to the active ingredient—a condition called *tachyphylaxis*. (I've had more than one patient tell me that their flaking scalp couldn't possibly be dandruff, since a dandruff shampoo didn't clear it up, when in fact the shampoo worked very well until tachyphylaxis took over.)

It's a good idea to avoid antidandruff products made with coal tar. Although these shampoos are better at controlling heavy scaling, they're also more likely to irritate sensitive scalp skin and should be used as a last resort. (Another disadvantage of coal tar preparations is their tendency to leave a greenish tinge on blond and light brown hair.)

If antidandruff shampoos made without coal tar don't bring significant improvement within six weeks or so, if your scalp is inflamed, or if there is heavy crusting, you may be wrestling with a case of seborrheic dermatitis. See a dermatologist. He or she might decide to okay use of a coal tar shampoo (but not if there is inflammation). Other courses of treatment could involve the use of cortisone gels, solutions, or sprays or, in severe cases, oral medication.

6

Remedies for Your Extremities: Stronger, Prettier Nails

I can't remember ever having a patient make an appointment to see me just because her nails were weak or brittle or discolored; the subject tends to come up in passing, after we've talked about the rash or the wrinkles or the hair loss or the acne. Nevertheless, it comes up often.

There's no denying the appeal of strong, healthy, well-groomed nails. How to get them—including what to do about common, minor nail problems—is what this chapter is all about. You'll also learn some useful tips to help you fake perfection, temporarily, when the occasion demands it.

Fragile Nails

Everyone wants nails that are strong enough and flexible enough to bend somewhat without breaking, chipping, or cracking. Strengthening them, if indeed they *can* be strengthened—some of us are just born with weak nails—can take months.

A good diet supplying adequate amounts of all the essential nutrients is crucial to your health and your appearance. But except in extreme cases, brittle, weak nails are rarely a consequence of what you eat or don't eat. Nails, like hair, are made of keratin, a protein, but getting more protein into your diet won't strengthen your nails unless you are suffering from a rather severe protein deficiency—not likely, unless you've been on a crash diet, are a strict vegetarian, or are anorexic.

In many instances weak nails are inherited. Sometimes nails weaken and become less flexible as a result of physical problems such as osteoporosis, iron deficiency anemia, thyroid irregularities, and conditions that impair circulation. If you're past menopause, weak nails could be a result of hormonal and other changes that have taken place in your body.

Brittleness can be caused by exposure to substances that dry out the nails. These include household cleaners and detergents, chemicals such as paint and varnish remover, and some nail polish removers.

"Toughening" Up Fragile Nails

Even when nails are inherently weak or have become less flexible as a result of physical ailments or menopause, there are a number of things you can do to encourage greater resilience. Don't look for overnight changes. It may be weeks or even months before you see improvement.

• Give your nails a "stronger" shape by filing them down so that they extend no more than about one-eighth inch past the tips of your fingers, rounding them slightly at the sides. Short, squarish nails may be less glamorous than long, tapered ones, but they break less easily. And squaring them off may make it possible for you to maintain all ten at a uniform length.

• Apply polish with built-in hardening ingredients, or use a brush-on nail hardening product.

IMPORTANT: Itchiness or redness could be a reaction to formaldehyde, a chemical ingredient in many nail hardeners. If irritation occurs, remove the product immediately, wait a few days, then look for a nail hardener made without formaldehyde, such as Clinique's Daily Nail Saver.

• Moisturize nails at bedtime. First get them good and wet with a ten-minute soak in warm water. (If you bathe in the evening, you can, of course, skip a separate soak for nails.) Blot up excess moisture, then massage petroleum jelly into each nail and the cuticle surrounding it. Rub it on hands, too, if they're dry. Put on an old pair of cotton gloves and wear them overnight.

• Try buffing, which promotes greater resiliency by stimulating circulation under the nails. You'll need a good buffer made of chamois and a buffing cream or powder, available at department stores and well-stocked drugstores. Instructions that come with the product will tell you how much cream or powder to use. Buff lightly and evenly over the entire nail surface. Since even very light buffing thins nails by removing upper cell layers, don't buff too often. Once a week is enough if your nails are thick. Average nails should be buffed less often. If your nails are very thin, you probably shouldn't buff at all.

• Wear cotton-lined gloves for dishwashing, hand laundering, and other wet work and whenever you must work with chemicals of any kind.

• Don't go out into the cold without gloves. Blustery weather can be just as drying to nails as to hands.

• Avoid frequent use of polish remover. Though it's a good idea to reinforce fragile nails by wearing polish with nail-hardening ingredients, it's not a good idea to change colors often, each time using a polish remover. Acetone, an ingredient in almost all removers, tends to dry nails, making them brittle and more likely to peel or break. Find a color you like and stick to it. When possible, make touch-up polish repairs instead of doing a whole new manicure. When you must remove polish, use an oily polish remover.

Splits and Tears

Even strong, healthy nails are not immune to splitting and tearing, but the problem is worse when nails are weak. With quick action, most small splits can be mended.

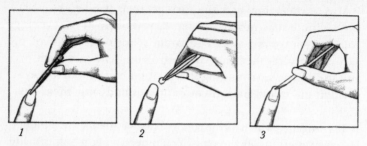

After placing a dot of glue on the area to be repaired (1), apply patching material (2), then press down and smooth with an orange stick (3).

Nail glue is the key. Keep some with your manicure tools. In a pinch you can use an instant household glue such as Krazy Glue. The ingredient that ensures quick, strong bonding—ethyl cryanoacrylate—is the same in both. You'll also need tweezers, a very fine emery board, a nail buffer, and a patch. Professional manicurists use very thin, fine-woven silk or linen for patching. Strong, thin paper, such as the kind used for teabags, is a good second choice. (To simplify, get a nail-mending kit containing patching material and adhesive; these are available at pharmacies and department stores.)

1. As soon as possible after you notice damage to your nail, snip patching material to a size and shape slightly larger than the area to be reinforced.

2. Squeeze a tiny dot of glue onto the torn portion of the nail. For a neater-looking repair, try not to overlap torn edges. Instead, nudge them together with tweezers.

3. Pick up fabric or paper patch with tweezers and place over the torn area. Dot on more glue. With an orange stick, gently smooth and press down loose edges of the patch.

4. Wait until glue is completely dry, then smooth away roughness with an emery board. Finish smoothing with the buffer.

5. Apply two coats of colored polish. (Only colored polish will hide the repairs.)

TIP: Always carry a Band-Aid in your purse. When you're away from home and a nail begins to tear, you can protect it with the Band-Aid and prevent damage from worsening.

No matter how careful you are, if you use your hands at all, your nails *will* occasionally chip, split, or tear. With care, though, you can reduce the incidence of these minor mishaps:

• Whenever possible, use a tool instead of your nails. To open a pop-top can, for example, insert a table knife under the lift-off tab; if you don't have a push-button phone, use the end of a pencil for dialing. When there's no tool suited to the job, work with the balls of your fingers, not the tips.

• Keep your nails relatively short. The less they extend beyond fingertips, the less there will be to snag and get caught on things.

• When you shape your nails, don't file down the sides too much. Slight rounding at the sides provides a stronger base.

Ridges and Grooves

To minimize the appearance of horizontal or vertical "ruts" in your nails, you'll need a buffer and a commercial ridge filler—a brush-on product that helps even out the surface of the nail. (These products are available at most drug- and variety stores.) The following procedure should make deeper grooves less noticeable, and very shallow grooves may disappear completely.

1. Lightly buff nails, from cuticles to tips, then from side to side, and again from cuticle to tip.

2. Rinse hands and nails in clear water. Dry thoroughly. Then apply ridge filler according to package instructions.

3. When ridge filler is dry and hard, apply two coats of colored polish.

Ridges and grooves are not an indication of dietary deficiencies, as many people believe. Rather, they are caused by trauma, to the nail itself, to the *nail bed*, which is the area directly under the visible part of the nail, or to the *matrix*, where the nail is "born." (The matrix is beneath the skin and begins almost as far back as the first joint of the finger.) When injury occurs to any of these areas—as, for example, when you accidentally hit your thumb with a hammer—the result can be bruising and/or slight deformity of the nail, such as a groove or ridge. Even pushing cuticles back too far or filing too vigorously can inflict damage that shows up later as a ridge. Inflammation of the nail bed, the cuticle area, or the matrix is another possible cause of ridges and grooves.

Time takes care of horizontal ridges. As the nail grows, the damaged area moves closer and closer to the tip until it reaches the file-off point. Vertical ridges, however, are sometimes an unavoidable consequence of growing older. When that is the case, they are more or less permanent.

If you are young and grooves or ridges appear frequently and for no apparent reason, see a dermatologist. The problem might be due to some underlying, treatable condition.

Discoloration

Yellowish or brownish stains are often traces of polish pigment embedded in the nail. (Very bright and very deep shades are most likely to stain.) Don't scrub at these stains with polish remover. It won't work, and it's too hard on nails. Try gentle buffing instead; light staining should come off along with topmost cell layers. If buffing doesn't work, and if your nails are thick and strong, you can try "sanding" stains with a very fine-grained emery board. Bleaching with lemon juice is sometimes recommended for removing stains from nails. There's no harm in wiping discolored areas with a cloth saturated with the juice of a lemon, but you'll find that lemon juice doesn't have enough bleaching power to lighten any but the faintest stains. The slowest but surest cure is to allow stains to fade gradually, by going without polish for a few weeks.

To prevent future staining of this type, apply one or two base coats of clear polish before brushing on color. The base coats will act as a barrier, preventing pigment from penetrating the nail.

A dark purplish or black spot is almost always dried blood—a scab—that has formed under the nail on the nail bed, and is the result of an injury severe enough to cause bleeding. If you're lucky, the scab will slowly disintegrate and fade away. Often, though, a scab under a nail will cause the nail to loosen, lift from its bed, and eventually fall off. If it looks as if you're going to lose a nail, don't do anything to hasten the process. Let it happen naturally. New growth is already well under way in the matrix, and it won't be long before there is enough to cover the bare nail bed. Don't polish and don't apply a fake nail over an infant nail still in the formative stage. Wait at least until it has grown long enough to cover the quick.

Spotty darkening and/or loss of translucency sometimes occurs with age. Opaque polish is the only remedy for this kind of discoloration.

A white spot indicates that a nail has separated and lifted from its bed. When there is only one small spot that moves toward the tip of the nail as the nail grows, the spot is probably the result of minor trauma. Cover it up with opaque polish if it bothers you. A number of white spots can indicate a dietary insufficiency of calcium or zinc.

Have a dermatologist take a look at a spot of *any* color if it appears to be getting larger, if the nail itself seems to be thickening and feels moist, and/or if there is soreness or inflammation of the nail or surrounding skin. Any of these point to a possible fungus infection.

Hangnails

These aren't nails at all, of course, but "tags" of torn skin hanging loose at the side or root of a nail. There is no quick and easy way to fix a hangnail, but you may be able to speed healing and minimize further tearing, which could lead to pain and infection:

1. Wash your hands. Then, with small, very sharp scissors, carefully clip off the dead, dry *tip* of the hangnail.

2. Apply an antibacterial ointment, such as Bacitracin, on the area, and cover with an adhesive strip. The strip will help prevent snagging and remind you not to pick.

Keep in mind that hangnails occur more often when skin is dry. If you are bothered by frequent hangnails, do the following:

• Wear cotton-lined rubber gloves when you work with liquids and when you must handle chemicals such as paint, solvents, furniture polish.
• Keep a bottle of hand lotion near the sink and use it every time you wash your hands.
• Rub petroleum jelly into cuticles and nails at night.

Ragged Cuticles

In looking at beauty books and magazine articles, I've noticed that they all tell readers to push back cuticles before applying nail polish. But they never tell how. Done improperly, the procedure can result in ragged, torn skin and hangnails. Here's the right way:

You'll need a good pair of cuticle clippers. Because clipper blades are designed to meet exactly, resulting in a clean, precise cut, these special tools are far better for cuticles than the sharpest manicure scissors. (The latter have overlapping blades and can pull and tug at skin.) Good clippers cost $10 and up, but the investment will be worth it if you do your own nails most of the time.

1. Soak hands in warm, sudsy water for about five minutes, then pat dry.

2. Wrap the end of a clean cloth or dish towel around the index finger of your right hand and gently nudge back cuticles

of thumb and fingers of your left hand. Repeat, gently pushing back cuticles of your right hand. (Don't use a bath towel for this; it's too heavy and you won't be able to feel what you're doing.)

3. If cuticles refuse to budge, apply a cuticle remover. Use according to instructions on the label.

4. Wipe away cuticle remover. Then gently insert the tapered end of an orange stick under the cuticle and slide it along, carefully lifting the yellowish edge from the nail. Do *not* poke or prod the stick past the loosened, dead cuticle and into the pink skin behind it. If you meet with resistance, soak for a few more minutes and try again.

5. Clean cuticle clipper blades with a cotton ball dipped in rubbing alcohol. Then work your way slowly and carefully around each nail, nipping off dead yellowish skin only and leaving a thin, neat rim of pink skin framing the nail. It's better to nip off too little dead skin than too much. (The pink skin around nails is "alive"; clipping into it might result in bleeding, soreness, even infection.)

TIP: Gently push cuticles back as a matter of course after each bath or shower and they'll be easier to deal with when you manicure your nails. If you push them back regularly, overgrown cuticles may also gradually begin to recede slightly, exposing more of the "moon" and making your nails look longer.

Bitten Nails

I don't have to tell you they're an eyesore and that once ingrained, the nail-biting habit is hard to break. There are bitter-tasting liquids which, when applied to fingertips, supposedly discourage biting. Frankly, I've never known anyone who stopped as a result of using one of these products. Maybe you'll be the exception.

More helpful, I think, is to make a firm commitment to stop biting and to start taking care of your nails. Keep cuticles smooth and well groomed and nails free of ragged edges. (Carry an emery board with you *always* and smooth away roughness before you're tempted to chew it off!) A substitute activity, such as playing with worry beads, or even squeezing a soft rubber ball when hands are idle, has helped a couple of my patients become ex-nail biters.

Occasionally, a patient will ask about wearing press-on artificial nails as an aid to breaking the habit. I don't think it's a good idea, since leaving them on for more than a couple of days at a time can lead to problems. However, fake nails are okay for special occasions when you want to look your best. (For more about artificial fingernails, see pages 114–16.)

The Fifteen-Minute Manicure

The very best manicures are done by professionals. They know all the tricks, have an assortment of special tools in good working order, and don't have to be ambidextrous to do an equally good job on each hand. Still, with a little practice most women can give themselves a perfectly good manicure. The step-by-step procedure below is a quickie version passed along to me by a patient who's a manicurist at a top salon. If you have more than fifteen minutes, soak your hands and work on your cuticles (as described earlier), *after* removing old polish. If you are limited to a quarter of an hour, here's what to do:

1. Gather tools and supplies: oily polish remover, cotton balls, cotton swabs, emery boards, polish, a bowl full of ice water or some salad oil.

2. Wipe away old polish with a cotton ball saturated with polish remover. Wipe down the length of each nail, turn the cotton to expose a clean area, and wipe again. To clean away stubborn polish at the sides and along the cuticle, use a cotton swab dipped in polish remover. Finish one nail before moving on to the next.

3. Wash and thoroughly rinse your hands. Clean under nails and rims of cuticles with the wedge-shaped end of an orange stick.

4. Smooth nails with an emery board. Use the fine side of the board, hold it at an angle slightly under the edge of the nail, and with light, quick strokes "brush" from right side to center of nail. Repeat, working from left side to center. Finish off with long, light sweeping strokes to round off the tip.

5. Apply polish. If you are right-handed, start with the nails on your right hand. If you're left-handed, start with the left. (In starting with your "good" hand, it will be easier to work on the other hand without smearing the polish you've already applied.) Polish the pinky fingernail of either hand first and work inward, nail by nail, to the thumb.

If your polish tends to wear off quickly along the ends of your nails, polish the edges, and underneath the tip of the nail as well.

Do the nails of each hand as above. Neaten up smears on cuticle or skin with a cotton swab dipped in polish remover.

6. Wait about five minutes or until the last nail polished feels smooth, not sticky, when you lightly touch the tip of your tongue to it.

7. If you've got a few minutes to spare, brush on another coat of polish. Wait sixty seconds or so, then "set" it by plunging fingertips into a bowl of ice water. Or, if you prefer, dip a fresh cotton swab in a little salad oil and smooth lightly over your nails. It takes *hours* for nail polish to "cure"—that is, dry completely. Until then, it can be scratched or peeled off fairly easily. Ice water, salad oil, or a commercial quick-dry spray helps prevent smudging in the meantime.

Shapes and Colors for More Attractive Hands

More tips from my manicurist patient:

• Broad nails. To create the illusion of greater slimness, wear your nails long. Instead of rounding them off at the tips, shape them into classic ovals. Choose medium shades of polish, such as coral and true red. Don't apply polish across the full width of your nails: they'll seem narrower if you leave just a hairs-breadth of space color-free on each side.

• Short nails. If they're short because they break or chip easily, follow the guidelines for strengthening fragile nails. In the meantime, keep cuticles well groomed and pushed back as far as possible to reveal the moons and expose more nail. Don't try to do too much at once. It may take several weeks of gentle nudging to coax overgrown cuticles back far enough to un-cover the moons. ("Gentle" is the key word here; remember, overvigorous prodding might damage the matrix, causing ridges or other minor nail deformities.) Best polish colors for short nails are those that blend in with surrounding skin—soft, sandy pinks, pale, rosy beiges, and so on.

• Stubby fingers. Longish tapered nails can make pudgy fin-gers look narrower and more elegant. Wear polish that mimics your skin tone so that there's no obvious line of demarcation between finger and nail.

• Hooked and spooned (upward-curling) nails. Nails with a tendency to curl down or up cannot be "trained" to grow straighter. But since curling becomes more pronounced as nails grow longer, hooking or spooning can be minimized by keep-ing nails fairly short. (Nails that are spooned up at the base can be an indication of anemia.)

What You Should Know About Fake Nails

The obvious solution to many nail problems is to cover up or extend nails by artificial means. If the sales figures for fake nails, nail tips, wrapping, and extension kits mean anything, millions of women are doing just that. Millions more are hav-ing their nails wrapped or extended in salons. But just because so many others are wearing them doesn't mean artificial nails are appropriate problem-solvers for you.

For one thing, if your real nails are weak and brittle, the adhesives and glues used to secure full fakes, tips, wraps, or extensions could very well weaken them further.

An even greater problem is the tendency of artificial nails to inhibit the evaporation of moisture. Water gets trapped underneath, and the area becomes a breeding ground for microorganisms and the development of a fungus infection—at its worst, red, swollen, pussy, very painful, difficult to treat, not to mention the fact that it can result in loss or permanent malformation of a nail.

I've had plenty of experience with fungus infections that seem to have gotten their start under an artificial nail of one kind or another. Unfortunately, when false nails are worn continuously, the infection, which first appears as a small dark spot, may be well under way by the time the patient becomes aware of it, making treatment even more difficult. The problem is compounded if the patient's job requires frequent hand washing or other work with liquids. One woman, a nurse, with a particularly resistant infection, actually had to take a leave of absence from her job at a hospital to give the medication a chance to clear up the fungus infection under her thumbnail.

Obviously, I'm not a fan of false nails. That doesn't stop my patients from wearing them, and it probably won't stop you, either. If you feel you must wear them, take the following precautions:

• Save artificial nails for special occasions. Don't wear them on the job if you're a waitress, bartender, nurse, doctor, or work in some other capacity that involves frequent immersing of your hands in water or other liquids. Remember, false nails tend to trap moisture and set up an ideal situation for the growth of fungi and other microorganisms.
• Do not wear artificial nails of any kind for more than forty-eight hours at a time. Following this guideline means you'll be limited to fakes that are fairly easy to remove. The easiest to apply and take off are full-size nails (as opposed to tips) secured with adhesive tabs. These can also be reused. Nail wraps and sculpted nails meant to be worn until the natural nail grows out are more difficult to apply, more expensive, more difficult to take off, and not reusable once they've been removed.
• Be alert to signs of irritation. If redness, itchiness, soreness,

or stinging develop while you're wearing false nails, remove them immediately. Do not reapply the nails until irritation subsides. If irritation returns after applying nails a second time, don't force the issue. You are hypersensitive or allergic to the adhesive, or to something in the nails themselves, and should not wear them. If redness or some other abnormality persists for more than two or three days after you've stopped wearing the nails, see a dermatologist.

• Do not apply false nails if any of your own nails appear to have thickened, seem moist or sore, or if you notice a dark spot (other than one you know to be a bruise). Any of these symptoms could indicate the presence of a fungus infection and should be watched closely. If there is no improvement within two or three days, see a dermatologist.

On Your Toes

The tips for keeping fingernails healthy and strong work for toenails too. To correct or minimize brittleness, ridges, discoloration, and so on, try the appropriate remedies and preventive measures given earlier in this chapter.

Your toes, including nails, matrix, nail bed, cuticle, and surrounding skin, are just as vulnerable to potential irritants and allergens as are your fingers—perhaps more so, considering the closed-in, damp "environment" provided by stockings and shoes. Reactions to polish are not common, but if you notice irritation, redness, soreness, or swelling soon after a pedicure, remove the polish and wait a few days to see what happens. Check with a dermatologist if the condition remains the same or worsens.

Tough Toenails

Despite the similarities of fingernails and toenails, some problems are more likely to affect one or the other. Extreme thickening is a more common problem in toenails. Abnormally thick nails often turn dark, take on a rough, bumpy texture, and curl downward as they grow. Friction and pressure from shoes that rub up against the tips of toes are factors that can cause toe-nails to grow so thick and tough they are almost impossible to trim. (Heredity and age are other factors; most of the people who see me about this condition are well into middle age, though I have one young patient, a fifteen-year-old girl, with this problem.)

When a thickened nail reaches a certain length, it usually loosens and drops off of its own accord. What remains of the nail is often near normal in thickness, color, and texture, but gradually thickens up again if it is not kept short by trimming every few days.

If a toughened toenail grows long enough to cause discomfort or embarrassment yet shows no sign of loosening and falling off on its own, try trimming it as follows. You'll need a large bowl or basin of warm, sudsy water, emery boards, and a good pair of toenail clippers.

1. Stroke the coarse side of an emery board several times back and forth across the *top* of the downward-curling tip of the nail. The object is to thin the nail by taking off some of the upper cell layers.

2. Soak your feet for ten minutes, then blot dry with a towel.

3. With the clippers, take small, angled "bites" from the tip of the nail. To avoid splitting or cracking the nail, do not attempt to clip straight across it.

4. Continue to clip off small angled portions of the nail tip, gradually shortening it to approximately normal length. Neaten the edge with the coarse side of an emery board; switch to the fine side to remove remaining roughness.

5. If the surface of the nail is rough-textured and dark, you can try "erasing" roughness and discoloration with the coarse side of an emery board. Use light strokes and do not take off too much of the surface.

Remember, if you keep nails short and wear roomy shoes that do not crowd your toes, it may not be necessary to repeat the procedure described above.

This method of dealing with toughened, discolored nails works in many cases. But some are so thick, they really need the attention of a dermatologist or podiatrist. If thinning and soaking as described seem to be getting you nowhere, don't force the issue. Take the problem to a professional.

Ingrown Toenails

There's no instant fix for a toenail that, instead of growing properly, has turned under and forced itself into the skin at the side or end of a toe. But it may not be necessary to seek medical treatment if you take steps to "reroute" the nail before it penetrates too deeply into skin.

If a nail is only *slightly* ingrown, place a tiny wad of sterile cotton between nail and flesh. (I instruct patients to insert it gently, with a toothpick.) This helps encourage the nail to straighten out and protects skin as well. Be sure to replace the old cotton with fresh after each shower or bath. Do keep an eye on the condition, though, and if the nail persists in growing improperly, see a doctor.

IMPORTANT: Even when ingrowth is very slight, don't attempt self-treatment if there is pain or soreness, redness, swelling, drainage (serum or pus), or bleeding in the area. Get medical attention immediately.

Toenails are less likely to become ingrown when they are clipped straight across. Don't shape them into ovals or round them at the sides. It's also important to wear shoes with plenty of toe-room.

Pedicure Pointers

A pedicure is very similar to a manicure, except for two important differences: Toenails should never be shaped, only clipped or cut straight across; cuticles should be coaxed back just enough to make feet look neat and well cared for, never trimmed.

The Forty-Five-Minute Pedicure

1. Remove old polish.
2. Soak your feet in warm soapy water for ten to fifteen minutes. Then pat dry.
3. Smooth callused areas with a pumice stone or foot file, presoaked in water. For better results with these tools, use a brisk but gentle circular motion instead of scraping back and forth.
4. Gently push cuticles back toward the base of the nails with the wedge-shaped end of an orange stick. Then clean around and under cuticles with the pointed end.
5. Trim nails with toenail clippers if you have them. (These are slightly larger than the clippers used for fingernails.) Remember, nails should be cut straight across. Use an emery board to smooth sharp edges at corners, but do not file down into the sides of nails. As for length, toenails should extend only to the ends of toes. When longer, not only do they look unkempt, but problems, such as ingrowing, can arise from the pressure or friction of a nail rubbing against the fronts of shoes (or even tight stockings!).
6. To counter dryness, massage body or hand lotion onto soles, tops of feet, toes, and ankles.
7. Use a cotton ball or swab dampened with polish remover to clean away traces of lotion on nails. Apply at least two coats of polish (three would last longer), allowing about five minutes' drying time between coats. To prevent polish from smearing onto adjacent toes, separate them with wads of tissue.
8. To speed final drying, you can dunk your feet into ice water, apply salad oil with a cotton swab, or use a nail polish drying spray. Even these speed-setting tricks won't prevent smearing if you get into stockings and shoes too soon after a pedicure, so wait at least an hour, if possible, before dressing.

7

Rashes, Redness, Itches, Bumps

Have you ever been puzzled by a rash, blotchy redness, welts, tiny blisters, or other sudden small skin problem and dismayed by what it did to your appearance? Of course you have. (Sooner or later, one or more of these nuisances get to everyone.) Most of these fall into the now-you-see-them, now-you-don't category, particularly if they are treated properly and promptly.

Please keep in mind that the following self-help measures should be used only when a problem is localized, not chronic, and unaccompanied by fever or pain. See a doctor about any rash, redness, blisters, or welts that cover large areas of your body, appear to be infected, are painful to the touch, or occur in conjunction with symptoms of physical illness.

Blotches

Pink or reddish blotchiness, with or without a warm, flushed "prickly" sensation, is a result of increased blood flow to the surface of the skin. Common causes include exposure to certain cosmetic ingredients, eating highly spiced food, drinking alcoholic beverages, vigorous exercise, and indoor or outdoor temperature extremes. Blotchiness is seen most often in people whose skin is thinner and more sensitive than average.

Any of the following treatments should help relieve blotchiness. However, if your skin tends to be oily, you might obtain somewhat speedier relief if you use the method designated for oily or combination skin. The dry-skin treatment is the gentlest of the three and a good choice if your skin is dry and quite sensitive.

A Quick Calm-Down for Blotchy Skin

1. Wash your face with lukewarm water and mild soap. Use your fingertips, not a washcloth.

2. Brew some chamomile tea or steep a chamomile tea bag in a cup of hot water for a few minutes.

3. When tea has cooled to skin temperature, saturate a clean cloth or cotton balls in it, wring out excess, and press gently to your face. Repeat applications for ten minutes.

4. Pat your face dry. If necessary, brew more tea and treat again in four hours.

How to Relieve Blotchiness on Oily or Combination Skin

1. Wash your face with lukewarm water and mild soap. Don't use a washcloth. Rinse thoroughly and pat dry.

2. Dip a cotton ball into Burow's Solution (available in drugstores prediluted or in packets to be diluted according to label instructions.) Press out excess and pat gently on blotchy areas. Repeat several times.

3. Pat your face dry and repeat the treatment in four hours, if necessary.

Keep your hands off your face for the next few hours. Don't wash again; don't use acne medication, astringents, or other drying products. Don't wear foundation. If you must wear makeup, limit it to hypoallergenic lipstick, eye shadow, and perhaps mascara.

How to Relieve Blotchiness on Dry Skin

1. Wash with lukewarm water and mild soap. (If your skin is very dry and sensitive, use a gentle soapless cleanser formulated for sensitive skin. I often recommend Lowila or Keri Facial Cleanser.) Rinse by splashing with lukewarm water and pat dry.

2. Apply a light-textured soothing lotion such as Nutraderm. Pat it on very gently. Don't rub it in.

3. Reapply lotion every four hours if necessary.

Touch your face as little as possible for the next several hours. Don't wash again. Don't apply makeup unless you feel it is absolutely necessary. If that's the case, skip foundation and wear only hypoallergenic lipstick, eye shadow, and mascara.

Itchy Red Rashes

When your skin reddens and turns itchy, think back over the last few hours and try to remember if you've been exposed to anything out of the ordinary. If there's any possibility that you've come into contact with poison ivy, don't waste a single second. Turn immediately to the poison ivy section on page 132. If it's hot out and you've been perspiring heavily, the problem might be heat rash. See page 131. Have you been handling detergents or household chemicals? The itchy redness might be a reaction to one of them. If so, you'll want to identify the irritant or allergen; more about that later. For now, here's what you can do, yourself, to get quick, safe relief.

How to Ease Itchy Redness on Face or Hands

1. Wash the affected areas with a soapless cleanser such as Lowila. Rinse thoroughly and pat dry.

2. Smooth on a 0.5 percent hydrocortisone cream, available without a prescription at drugstores.

3. Reapply hydrocortisone cream every four hours if necessary.

Easing a Rash on Other Body Areas

1. Run warm, not hot, water into the bathtub. As the tub is filling, add a colloidal oatmeal product, such as the one made by Aveeno. (For even dispersion, sift it in with a flour sifter.) Settle into the tub and soak. After fifteen to twenty minutes, get out and pat dry with a clean, soft towel.

2. Apply an over-the-counter 0.5 percent hydrocortisone cream to affected areas.

3. Reapply the cream every four hours if necessary.

More Itch Relief

Hydrocortisone cream is often enough to ease itchiness. But if you need extra help, try the following:

• Apply a cold or hot compress. A convenient no-drip way to "freeze out" an itch is to crush some ice cubes, place them in a plastic sandwich bag, and hold it against the affected area for a few minutes.

To apply heat, you can use a clean washcloth or a corner of a towel that has been dipped into hot water and wrung out. (Be careful. Make sure the compress has cooled enough not to burn your skin.) Or try a gel-type thermal pack, which picks up heat when immersed in hot water. Sold in drugstores primarily to ease backache and the soreness associated with muscle injuries, these packs are handy whenever heat is called for, since they retain warmth for longer periods than a cloth compress. (Once again, be careful not to burn yourself. For safety's sake, place the hot pack between two folded towels.)

• Take an oral antihistamine, such as Chlor-Trimeton or Benadryl. Of course, as with all over-the-counter preparations, make a point of reading the label and instructions, including precautionary information, if any.

Identifying Irritants and Allergens

Redness, itching, and swelling can be the result of contact with an irritant or an allergen. In some cases, onetime exposure to an irritating substance causes an almost-instant reaction. In other cases, the skin reacts to frequent or prolonged contact with irritating substances. When it comes to allergies, a reaction usually occurs after at least two exposures to the allergen. The first contact sensitizes the skin and causes changes that result in flare-ups on future contact with the troublemaker.

Reactions can range from a slight pinkish tint with little or no itch to an angry red inflammation accompanied by a raging urge to scratch. If there is continued exposure to the irritant or allergen, and if the condition goes untreated, it can progress to blistering, crusting, scaling, and worse.

Obviously, it makes sense to try to identify the offending substance at the first sign of trouble so that future problems can be avoided. This may take a bit of detective work, since almost anything can spark a reaction. Some substances are more likely to cause problems than others, though. These are the ones that belong at the top of any suspect list.

Prime Cosmetic Suspects

In my experience, the worst offenders are quaternary ammonium compounds (especially quaternium 15). These compounds are ingredients in many of the preservatives, germicides, sanitizers, and antiseptics used in formulating a variety of deodorants and antiperspirants, after-shave lotions, regular and antidandruff shampoos, cuticle removers, hairstyling, coloring, and waving products, and other toiletries.

Formaldehyde is also near the top of the cosmetic suspect list. The chemical is found in some soaps and hair preparations as well as in many nail products, including polish and nail hardeners. Reactions to these can be severe and include discoloration, bleeding, even loss of a nail; the cuticle and surrounding skin might also be involved.

Quaternium 15 and formaldehyde are among the most common cosmetic causes of contact dermatitis and are known eye irritants.

Of the following likely offenders cited by the North American Contact Dermatitis Group (which is affiliated with the American Academy of Dermatology), fragrances and preservatives are the most common:

acrylate
fragrances
glyceryl monothioglycolate
lanolin and its derivatives
methacrylate
PABA, found in many sunscreens
p-Phenylenediamine
preservatives and antibacterial agents
propylene glycol
toluenesulfonamide

To track down the cause of a rash, try to remember what new and even not-so-new cosmetics or toiletries you've been using on the affected areas of your skin.

A rash on the face? Your cleanser, moisturizer, toner, astringent, blusher, lipstick, and other makeup are all suspects. Hair dye, permanent-wave and curl-relaxing solutions can cause problems on the face as well as on the scalp, as can shampoo, conditioner, hairspray, mousse, setting lotions, and gels. A body rash can be triggered by perfume, cologne, toilet water, and other fragrance products, deodorants, sunscreens, tanning lotions, bath salts or crystals, soaps, and so on.

Cosmetics and toiletry ingredients are printed on the package or container in descending order of proportion, so check these listings to see if any of the substances on the above suspect list are present in the products you use. If so, you may have identified the villain.

Tɪᴘ: Fragrance allergies are not unusual. However, the individual ingredients that make up a particular fragrance are not listed on labels. Thus it's impossible to pinpoint and avoid specific substances. If you suspect fragrance is responsible for a rash, your best bet is to avoid all perfumes and scented products and to use instead those labeled "fragrance free" or "unscented."

When in doubt about the cause of a rash on face or body, don't use *any* cosmetics or personal care products for a few days. Then test each preparation before you use it again, by dabbing a small amount inside the bend of your elbow. Cover with a bandage and wait at least twenty-four hours to see if a rash or other irritation develops. Do the same when trying new products. And to be on the safe side, don't try more than one new product at a time.

I also advise my patients to use products with the fewest number of ingredients, since these products are least likely to cause problems. After all, the longer the ingredient list for a product, the greater the number of potential troublemakers it contains. This is as true of a lipstick or nail polish as it is of the latest high-tech moisturizing formulation.

If your skin tends to be easily irritated, you might want to consider switching to cosmetics and toiletries labeled "hypoallergenic" or "allergy tested," such as those formulated by Almay, Bonne Bell, Physicians Formula, and Clinique, among others. Neither term, incidentally, guarantees that a product is entirely free of all potential allergens; however, it is an indication that an attempt has been made to eliminate or reduce the amount of some of the most common offenders.

Other Irritants and Allergens

Cosmetics and toiletries aren't the only potential troublemakers. Almost any substance or material can irritate or ignite an allergic reaction. But some tend to cause more problems than others. Included among these are:

alcohol
bathroom cleansers
bleaches
car waxes and polishes
chalk
citrus fruit
detergents and soaps
furniture and floor waxes and polishes
gasoline
hot water
lacquers
lighter fluid
nickel
paints and paint thinners
raw meat
rubber
solvents
some vegetables, including garlic, potatoes, onions, okra
urine on diapers and in diaper pails

Of all the potential irritants and allergens, nickel is the most common. It's so common it deserves special attention here.

Nickel, Public Allergy Number One

A rash on earlobes, front and back; a disk-shaped rash on the wrist; a rash that encircles your finger—any of these point to a nickel allergy. This metal is an ingredient in many alloys used in the manufacture of watches, earrings, rings, and other jewelry (even some "good" jewelry; small amounts of nickel may be present in gold, silver, and platinum). It's also used in many metal buttons, snaps, belt buckles, some zippers, hairpins and hair ornaments, as well as in numerous items found in the home and office. Nickel, in short, is omnipresent.

There is evidence that some nickel allergies are initiated by ear piercing, which can sensitize the earlobes and eventually other parts of the body. In some cases, at least, the allergy might be prevented if ears are pierced with a stainless steel needle and only earrings with stainless steel posts are worn thereafter.

But what if you're already allergic to this metal? There are several things you can do to prevent or minimize contact—and the itchy red rashes that can result.

• Don't wear metal jewelry. If my patients' horrified reaction to this advice is any indication, few women are willing to give up metal jewelry altogether. If you're one of them, do the next best thing. Apply to the back of your favorite metal jewelry several coats of clear nail polish. (Allow ample drying time between coats.) The polish will act as a barrier between you and the metal, preventing direct contact. Frequently worn jewelry will require recoating from time to time.

• In the future, purchase only earrings with stainless steel posts or those labeled "hypoallergenic."

• Avoid using clips, hairpins, barrettes, and other hair ornaments made of metal. Look for plastic or wood alternatives.

• Replace metal buttons, zippers, et cetera, with plastic, bone, wood.

• Cover with adhesive tape metal doorknobs, dials, and the handles of tools, cutlery, pots, pans, and other items you must use frequently.

Hand Rashes

Because they're exposed to so many irritants—including but not limited to those listed on page 127—hands are especially vulnerable. Frequent immersion in hot water and detergent solution (which are irritants) makes hands even more sensitive and rash-prone. Pre-existing conditions such as psoriasis, allergy (atopic dermatitis), a bacterial or fungal infection may play a role in aggravating a hand rash. Often, what begins as a relatively minor problem can quickly turn into something more severe.

If the rash on your hands has been there for more than a week or so, if the skin is broken, blistered, or crusted, or has turned dark and leathery, see a dermatologist as soon as possible.

To ease a minor hand rash, do the following:

1. Repeated wetting and drying weakens the skin's natural defenses and makes hands more susceptible to irritants and allergens. For this reason, avoid or minimize contact with water except when treating your hands as below. When you must wash, use a mild soap or soap substitute. I often recommend Dove, Basis, Neutrogena Dry Skin Formula, Lowila, Oilatum, pHresh, or Alpha Keri soap.

2. After washing, shake off excessive moisture and apply a 0.5 percent hydrocortisone cream to damp skin. Pat dry with a towel and reapply cream.

3. When hands feel itchy, fill a bowl or bathroom basin with cold water and add a few drops of mild bath oil, such as Aveeno, Alpha Keri, Lubath, or Kauma. Immerse hands for several minutes, then smooth on hydrocortisone cream. Follow with a hand cream, such as Eucerin, Nivea, Aquacare Lotion, Purpose Dry Skin Cream, Ever Soft Skin Care Lotion, Aquaderm, Ultra-Rich Moisturizing Lotion, or Complex 15.

4. Apply hydrocortisone cream four times a day until rash disappears and skin returns to normal. For a month or so after that, continue to use the cream, gradually decreasing the number of applications per day. During the post-rash period, skin is still sensitive and needs special care.

5. Avoid direct contact with household cleaners, bleaches, and hot water. All of these can remove protective oils from the skin and interfere with its ability to retain moisture—a state that invites further problems.

6. When you must work with allergens and irritants, such as those listed on page 127, protect your hands with gloves. Wear thin white cotton "dermal" gloves (available at many pharmacies) when handling dry substances, cotton-lined rubber gloves when working with liquids. Sprinkle talc or cornstarch inside rubber gloves to absorb perspiration, and if possible, do not

wear them for more than half an hour since moisture can aggravate a rash. (Launder gloves to remove traces of perspiration before wearing them again.) If liquid seeps inside rubber gloves, remove them immediately and pull on a fresh, dry pair.

7. Gloves or no gloves, avoid immersing hands in very hot water.

Frankly, hand rashes are among the most frustrating and difficult-to-treat conditions a dermatologist runs up against. Patients want to get better and usually follow their doctor's recommendations to the best of their ability, but the fact that we all use our hands in so many ways all day, every day, tends to complicate treatment. It's not easy to keep hands out of water. It's a bother to have to put on gloves before touching certain foods and chemicals. And even when a patient does everything else right, he or she sometimes remains unaware that a particular substance may be aggravating the problem.

A patient of mine named Barbara saw a small improvement soon after she began treatment, but her hands quickly reverted to the red, raw, itchy state they were in when I first saw her. She followed all my recommendations. She used moisturizers and hydrocortisone cream exactly as I'd instructed. She wore gloves for wet work and food preparation, and even with gloves on, never put her hands in hot water. In fact, she assured me that she never used her bare hands to touch *anything* on the list of common irritants I'd given her on her initial visit to the office.

"Not even chalk?" I asked, remembering that Barbara was a schoolteacher and probably used chalk every day. It was a lucky guess. Though chalk is clearly listed on the suspect list, she (like some other patients I've known) had a hard time believing that something so seemingly innocuous could trigger a rash. Once she began to take precautions when handling chalk, we were able to clear up the condition. The point is that no matter how unlikely you think it might be that a certain substance or group of substances is responsible for a rash, if it's on the list, avoid it if possible. If you can't avoid it, wear gloves when you handle it. (Naturally, if something *not* on the list appears to be causing problems, avoid that, too.)

One more thing: If you've had one rash, consider yourself a prime candidate for future rashes. Even after your hands have returned to normal, continue to protect them: Keep them out of hot water. Wash, rinse, and apply plenty of moisturizer after immersion in liquids. Wear gloves when washing dishes, handling diapers, doing housework, working with paints and other chemicals, and preparing foods on the list of common troublemakers. And of course avoid contact with any substance that seemed to initiate a previous reaction.

Heat Rash (Prickly Heat)

Clusters of tiny red bumps or blisters on your neck or concentrated in body folds (the bend of elbows and knees, between breasts, etc.) could be heat rash—especially if the weather is hot and humid and you've been perspiring freely.

Also called prickly heat, heat rash can occur any time conditions prevent perspiration from evaporating and the skin is bathed for extended periods in its own moisture. Friction and pressure aggravate the condition.

How to Soothe Heat Rash

1. Bathe with a soapless soap such as Aveenobar or Dove. Limit time spent in tub or shower to five minutes. Pat thoroughly dry with a clean, soft towel.

2. Apply calamine lotion to affected areas. Or make up a paste of baking soda and water, smooth it on, and allow it to dry on skin.

3. To ease itching, apply crushed ice in a plastic sandwich bag. If skin is sore rather than itchy, smooth on a light, water-based moisturizing lotion such as Aquaderm or Neutrogena Moisture (which will be even more soothing if you chill it beforehand).

The best way to deal with heat rash is to stay cool. Choose light, loosely woven clothing, preferably of natural fibers such as cotton, linen, or silk. These absorb moisture better than synthetics, which tend to trap and hold it against the skin. Don't wear tight collars, tight belts, lingerie that binds, form-fitting skirts or tops, all-polyester garments, or rubber or plastic sweatsuits.

Before getting into your clothes, dust yourself with cornstarch or cornstarch-based powder. From time to time during the day, take a few minutes to rinse, dry, and repowder sweated-up areas. It's very important not to allow perspiration to stay in contact with your skin.

Spend as much time as possible in air-conditioned environments. Don't sit in the sun. Avoid activities that cause you to perspire excessively.

Poison Ivy

Speed is of the essence in treating poison ivy.

If you can get to a shower within ten minutes of exposure to poison ivy, oak, or sumac, soap-and-water scrubbing may prevent itchy redness and blisters. If you can bathe within an hour, the severity and duration of the rash may be minimized.

Unfortunately, once you've been sensitized to the oily plant compounds that trigger the condition, an eruption can occur without direct contact. For example, a teenage girl who swore she never strayed off the walkways or the beaches of the ocean-side community where she and her family spent summers, a community notorious for poison ivy in the undergrowth, was apparently infected via her cat. A woman patient of mine probably picked up her winter case of poison ivy while rummaging through the garden tools in search of a snow shovel. Another patient's mysterious brush with the condition seems to have been a result of using a laundry marker (the plant from which its ink is made is biochemically similar to poison ivy).

Since eruptions can be triggered indirectly, it's not always

easy to tell whether itchy redness is, indeed, due to poison
ivy (or one of its relatives), or whether it's the result of contact with some other irritant or allergen. The following clues
should help:

• Poison ivy reactions usually occur first on exposed areas of
the body—on hands, bare arms, and, most commonly, bare legs.
The exception is when contamination results from wearing
clothing that has been in contact with the plant oils. In that
case, skin areas covered by the clothing will erupt first.

• The rash begins as localized redness, typically accompanied
by itching. If you have been directly exposed, breakouts may
appear initially as short, reddened streaks on the skin, the result of leaves brushing against you as you walk past.

• Tiny blisters erupt, usually within hours after the redness
appears.

There's not much you can do to protect yourself from indirect contamination—when plant oil residues are picked up
from a pet, gardening equipment, car or bicycle tires, and so
on. But you *can* avoid direct exposure by learning to recognize the plants and keep your distance. They're not difficult
to identify. Leaves are glossy and sprout from stems in groups
of three. (Remember the old warning, "Leaflets three, let
it be.")

Keep in mind that you can be infected by contact with *any*
part of the plant, at *any* time of year. Don't try burning poison
ivy to eliminate it from your garden; even smoke from burning
plants can carry enough of the oils along with it to incite an
eruption.

Here's what to do when you've been exposed:

1. Run, don't walk, to the nearest shower. Wash with plenty
of soap and water as hot as you can tolerate. While still in the
shower, carefully clean under your fingernails. (If you're away
from home in an area where there are no shower facilities, do

the next best thing: wash your hands, face, and other exposed areas, in that order.)

2. Follow up with additional soap-and-water showers every three or four hours for the next twenty-four hours.

3. After tending to yourself, launder the clothing you wore when you were exposed—including underwear, socks, and shoes. (Throw sneakers into the washing machine; clean leather shoes with a cloth that has been soaked in a strong detergent solution and wrung out.) To prevent recontamination of yourself, wear a long-sleeved top and gloves when you handle your clothes.

4. To reduce itching and inflammation, apply clean cloths saturated with Burow's Solution, which you can get at a drugstore. Leave the cloths in place for five or ten minutes. Repeat as needed. If you're out in the woods on a camping trip and Burow's Solution is unavailable, compresses made with a solution of powdered milk and water, or a solution of salt and water, should help.

5. Try an over-the-counter oral antihistamine, such as Chlor-Trimeton, for further relief of itch and inflammation.

6. At bedtime, or whenever itching starts to get the better of you, run tepid water into the tub, add several handfuls of oatmeal or baking soda, and soak. Allow the powdery residue to dry on your skin.

7. Treat itching and blisters near your eyes by patting with sterile gauze squares dampened with diluted boric acid.

8. When it's time to appear in public, smooth on a thin film of calamine lotion. (Be careful not to get any in your eyes.) It won't disguise redness and swelling, but it will make them less obvious and provide some relief from itching.

9. Don't scratch. It can lead to infection. To minimize potential harm from scratching during sleep, shorten and smooth your fingernails with an emery board.

10. If itching is unbearable; if blisters and swelling occur very near your eyes or genitals; if the inflammation is severe and doesn't show gradual improvement within a few days after the first flare-up, but seems to stay the same or get worse—see

a dermatologist. He or she can prescribe topical and oral medications that will reduce your discomfort and speed poison ivy on its way better than anything you can cook up at home or buy over the counter.

Hives (Urticaria)

Stinging or itchy red welts that gradually turn pale and then disappear are probably hives. Caused by a release of histamine just beneath the skin, hives are often the body's response to an allergen, though there is sometimes a psychological basis to the condition. Frequent or lingering flare-ups could be an indication of infection. Cystitis, sinusitis, tonsillitis, an abscessed tooth, even ringworm, for example, can keep a case of hives going for weeks or even months. When the infection is cleared up, the hives tend to disappear along with it.

How to Combat an Attack of Hives

1. Bathe the area with lukewarm water. (Very warm water can step up the release of histamines and make hives worse.) Pat dry with a clean towel.

2. Apply a soothing lotion, such as Nutraderm. Or dab with a cotton ball dampened with witch hazel. For maximum relief, pre-chill lotion or witch hazel.

3. Ease intense itching or stinging with an ice pack of crushed ice in a plastic sandwich bag.

4. Try an over-the-counter oral antihistamine such as Chlor-Trimeton or Benadryl. These sometimes reduce the discomfort associated with a breakout of hives.

5. Don't take aspirin. It can aggravate the condition. If you need an analgesic, take one containing acetaminophen, such as Tylenol.

A note about vitamin C: Though its effectiveness has not been proven, vitamin C is sometimes "prescribed" for hives.

Give it a try if you like. However, discontinue supplemental vitamin C immediately if hives seem to worsen.

Hives tend to clear up rapidly, often within a day. That's the good news. The bad news is that they're uncomfortable, spoil your looks, and tend to make unwanted return appearances.

Hive-prone people (often those with a personal or family history of hay fever, migraine headaches, or asthma) can be sensitive to any number of substances, even minuscule amounts of which can incite a reaction. Determining the cause—or causes—is easier than finding a needle in a haystack, but not much. Still, it's worth the effort:

Start by keeping records. Next time you have a hive attack, get out paper and pencil and jot down what you ate, drank, and took in the way of medication during the preceding few hours. If you used a new cosmetic or toiletry, make note of that, too, as well as any exposure you may have had to animals, dust, pollen, unfamiliar plants, or an unusually large number of plants. Also try to remember and describe your mental state before an eruption of hives. Were you anxious? Angry? Frustrated?

Eating certain foods can cause hives. Suspect something you ate if hives occur in conjunction with gastrointestinal disturbance (queasiness, upset stomach, diarrhea). Many cases of hives have been sparked by the following:

    anything made with wheat
    beef, pork
    cabbage
    chocolate
    citrus fruit, strawberries, bananas, grapes, pineapple
    coffee, tea
    eggs
    milk, cheese
    navy beans
    spices, especially curry
    tomatoes, pickles

NOTE: Alcohol appears to heighten allergic reactions in some people. You might find that a glass of orange juice at breakfast is harmless, whereas orange juice and vodka at cocktail time could cause problems.

Some food dyes and preservatives have also been implicated, as well as ingredients in root beer and sarsaparilla. Wintergreen and mint flavorings, including those used in cough drops, throat lozenges, and even menthol cigarettes have been known to trigger reactions.

Aspirin, penicillin, and tetracycline are among the drugs that make trouble for some.

Even with careful recordkeeping, you may not be able to track down the cause(s) of hives. But in time a pattern may reveal itself—if not to you, then to a dermatologist, should you decide to seek professional help.

When should you see a doctor if you have frequent, severe, or lingering hives? They are not only uncomfortable and disfiguring; they could point to a more serious problem. You should have a medical checkup, which might include blood tests, urinalysis, a sinus examination, X rays for chest and teeth, as well as allergy testing. Even if you are inclined to tough it out on your own, see a doctor *immediately* even for a single, acute case of hives if your eyelids and/or lips are affected or if hives invade your mouth or throat where they can interfere with breathing.

Bathers' Bottom

This annoying rash—often itchy, occasionally sore or stinging—made up of tiny pimples or blisters on the buttocks and surrounding areas, is the result of sitting around too long in a wet bathing suit (or any other wet clothes). Bathers' bottom can also erupt after prolonged immersion in a hot tub.

To Clear Up Bathers' Bottom

1. Shower with lukewarm water and pat dry.
2. With a clean cloth or cotton balls, dab rubbing alcohol or witch hazel on the area and allow skin to dry in air.
3. If the rash is sore rather than itchy, smooth on an over-the-counter antibiotic cream, such as Desitin.

If possible, stay out of the water for a few days to allow time for the rash to subside. And of course, next time you swim, change into a dry, clean bathing suit or dry clothes immediately after your dip.

Swimmers' Itch

The small reddish bumps on arms, chest, legs, and other areas not covered by a bathing suit are caused by microorganisms infesting many lakes and seashore areas.

To Relieve Swimmers' Itch and Bumps

1. Shower with soap and water. Pat dry with a clean towel.
2. Apply calamine lotion to affected areas.
3. If the itch persists, try a 0.5 percent hydrocortisone cream. Repeat every four hours if necessary.

You may be able to prevent future problems caused by these microscopic pests by stripping and showering with warm soap and water immediately after swimming in a lake or ocean. Follow with an allover brisk rubdown with witch hazel or other mild astringent.

Insect Stings and Bites

The initial "ouch" is the least of it. Itching, soreness, swelling, and—if you are one of those who are especially sensitive to the venom of certain insects—the serious, possibly lethal allergic reaction that can follow are the real problems.

IMPORTANT: If you know or even suspect that you are allergic to insect stings, speak to your doctor about getting a prescription for an emergency sting treatment kit, such as Ana-Kit, and take it with you on all outings. If you don't have a kit with you and are stung or bitten, get to a doctor immediately. If necessary, have someone take you to the emergency room of the nearest hospital. An over-the-counter asthma inhaler may provide temporary relief while you're on your way.

What to Do About Insect Stings and Bites

If you're not allergic, treat stings and bites this way:

1. For a bee sting, remove the barbed stinger and attached venom sac. Don't use tweezers; you'll get the stinger but not the sac, which will continue to release venom into your skin. Don't squeeze the area; you'll crush the sac and more venom will flow out. Instead, scrape off stinger and sac with a sterilized needle, clean fingernail, or dull knife.

2. If the sting or bite site is on your foot or leg, keep it elevated for a while.

3. Wash the area with soap and warm water. Pat dry.

4. Apply one of the following: a paste made with equal parts plain (unflavored) meat tenderizer and water; a paste made of baking soda and water; crushed ice in a plastic sandwich bag.

5. When initial soreness subsides, smooth calamine lotion on the affected area to reduce itching. An oral antihistamine such as Chlor-Trimeton can also be a help.

See a doctor if swelling, itching, or pain is severe and does not subside within a day or so. He or she may decide to prescribe an antihistamine or cortisone-based medication.

To guard against getting stung again, take a good insect repellent—and use it—when you go out on hikes, camping trips, and picnics. Some of the best repellents contain a chemical listed on the label as DEET (or diethyl toluamide). Use the product according to instructions on the label.

In addition, don't wear fragrance out of doors. In this case, fragrance includes soaps, lotions, and other sweet-scented toiletries as well as perfume, toilet water, and cologne.

Finally, don't wear shiny jewelry or bright-colored clothing. Bugs are attracted to both.

Sunburn

It should never happen. Now that we know beyond doubt that sun exposure is a prime factor in the development of certain kinds of skin cancer, and that it causes many of the skin changes previously thought to be "normal" and inevitable consequences of aging, there's no reason ever to go out of doors without first applying a broad-spectrum, high SPF (sun protection factor) product. (See Chapter 9 for more about the aging effects of sunlight and what you can do to prevent and even reverse some of them.)

However, let's assume you were inadvertently caught somewhere on a sandy beach or ski slope without sun protection. Parts of your body were exposed enough to result in damage to epidermal cells and blood vessels, causing swelling and leakage of blood from capillaries. In other words, you got sunburned. What do you do? It depends on how severe the burn.

How to Self-treat First-Degree Sunburn (Characterized by Pinkness or Redness, Warmth, and Pain)

1. Apply a cream or lotion containing camphor, phenol, or menthol (Noxzema is one). Alternate with cold compresses. To make a compress, place a handful of ordinary raw oatmeal, Aveeno Bath (a commercial oatmeal extract available at drugstores), or cornstarch in a large square of sterile gauze, clean cheesecloth, or any clean, loosely woven cotton fabric. Fold the

ends of the cloth, run cold water through it, and wring out excess moisture. Place compresses directly on affected areas. Repeat as often as needed to obtain relief.

2. Between applications of cream and compresses, ease discomfort by applying ice wrapped in a clean cloth, or a clean cloth dipped and wrung out of ice water, chilled milk, or chilled witch hazel.

3. If you need more relief than that provided by the measures suggested above, smooth on an over-the-counter hydrocortisone cream.

4. Take aspirin, if necessary, to reduce pain and swelling. Aspirin substitutes, such as Tylenol, are not effective in soothing sunburn discomfort.

5. If your face is affected, keep it well moisturized. Do not wear makeup until swelling has gone down and redness has faded to pink.

For the first few days after exposure, bathe once or twice a day in cool water to which you've added several handfuls of Aveeno Bath. Drink plenty of liquids—eight full glasses of water a day—to help replenish body fluids lost through skin dehydration. Stay as cool as possible. Remain indoors near a fan or in an air-conditioned room. (Warmth and especially perspiration can increase sunburn discomfort.) For more comfort at night, sprinkle cornstarch, talc, or powder on your sheets.

What to Do About Severe Sunburn

If your skin turns very red and there is significant swelling accompanied by oozing or blisters, your sunburn requires medical attention. See a dermatologist or other doctor. To prevent infection and other possible complications, you need more help than the measures above can provide, including, perhaps, prescription medications containing corticosteroids or indomethican. In some cases, hospitalization is required.

When you're back to normal, promise yourself to take proper

precautions in the future. That means limiting time spent in the sun and wearing broad-spectrum, high SPF sunscreens every single time you go outdoors, whatever the season, and even in cloudy weather. (See Chapter 9 for information on how to select a sunscreen.)

Athlete's Foot

You don't have to be a fitness freak to contract this typically itchy, sometimes scaly and inflamed condition that appears most often between and around the toes. The organism that causes it can be picked up almost anywhere, lie dormant in irritated or lacerated skin, and then, when conditions are right, proliferate into a full-blown case. Men are more likely to develop athlete's foot, but women are not entirely immune.

Since athlete's foot is sometimes difficult to distinguish from other reddened, itchy, scaly, or blistered conditions (such as eczema or psoriasis), my advice is not to attempt self-treatment. The wrong over-the-counter remedy could aggravate those other conditions. See a dermatologist before you do anything else about the itchy redness you think might be athlete's foot. There are some things you can do to *prevent* this unpleasant condition:

• Dry your feet thoroughly after every bath or shower, paying special attention to areas between the toes. Then dust with a cornstarch-based powder.
• Wear shoes that "breathe"—leather or canvas, for example, as opposed to synthetics, such as plastic and rubber, which trap moisture. (Rubber boots are fine for rainy days but get out of them as soon as possible when you come indoors.) Except when you're wearing open sandals, don't go without socks (preferably cotton) or hose, both of which absorb excess moisture.
• Avoid walking barefoot on wet floors.

There are hundreds, maybe thousands, of less common conditions that manifest themselves as rashy redness, itchiness, blisters, bumps, and so on, and all of them can spoil the way you look and feel. But most of these others require prompt professional attention, and since this book is about what you can do to solve your own beauty problems—safely and quickly—descriptions of them and the medical procedures used to treat them would be out of place here.

Some of these conditions look and feel in their initial stages like the less serious ones covered in this chapter. For this reason, I urge you to see a doctor about any problem that does not respond to self-treatment within a few days or that seems to be getting worse. The easy, self-help remedies suggested here and elsewhere in this book can be very effective—but not when you have a serious condition that requires the attention of a doctor.

8

From Calluses to Stretch Marks to Unwanted Hair: What to Do About Miscellaneous Beauty Blots

Much of what a dermatologist does for a living has to do with treating what I call "little uglies"—calluses, corns, moles, warts—as well as a number of other unaesthetic conditions such as excess hair and perspiration. Everyone has a few of these (usually) minor problems. In this chapter, I'll tell you which you can deal with on your own, and how, and what to do when a problem is beyond self-treatment.

Calluses

If you're on your feet at all, you have some thickening of the skin on the undersides of your toes, the balls of your feet, and around your heels. Calluses are protective. The buildup of toughened skin is your body's response to, and defense against, the friction and pressure your feet are subjected to as you go about your everyday activities. When calluses become large enough and rough enough to be unsightly, snag hosiery, and cause discomfort, however, you'll want to do something about them.

Seven-Day Plan for Smoother Feet

1. In the evening, run warm water into the bathtub or a large basin, lather up a mild soap to make suds, and soak your feet for ten minutes.

2. Rinse and pat your feet damp-dry. Then go over roughened, callused areas with a pumice stone or foot file. (These work better if presoaked for a minute.) Instead of back-and-forth rubbing, use a gentle, circular motion.

3. Rinse again and dry your feet thoroughly. Apply a sloughing product which rolls away dry, dead skin. (Dr. Scholl's Smooth Touch Buffing Cream is a good example.) Use the product according to instructions on the label.

4. Rinse your feet again, pat to damp-dry, and rub on a generous amount of inexpensive moisturizer (petroleum jelly is fine for this purpose). Get into a pair of old, clean socks and wear them overnight.

The treatment above, repeated every night for a week or so, should soften, smooth, and somewhat reduce the size of calluses. If you want to reduce them even further, try over-the-counter adhesive-backed callus and corn "plasters" premedicated with salicylic acid. These pads are applied and left on for a few days, after which softened, callused skin can be lifted off. I prefer them to the liquid callus and corn removers, which can drip or run onto surrounding, uncallused skin. Be sure to read and follow to the letter all instructions on label or package insert.

IMPORTANT: Attempting self-surgery with a razor blade or other sharp instrument is asking for trouble. Don't even think

about it. If calluses are overgrown and/or uncomfortable
enough to interfere with ease of movement, and if the home
treatment above does not bring improvement, have them pared
down by a dermatologist or podiatrist.

Corns

Like calluses, these smooth, hard, often reddened and sometimes painful bumps, appearing most frequently on tops of
toes, are caused by pressure or friction. In the case of corns,
however, the pressure is almost always caused by shoes that
don't fit properly. A slight malformation of the foot can exac-
erbate corns, if bony protrusions are in constant contact with
shoes or boots.

To combat corns, take the pressure off. Stop wearing shoes
or boots that crowd or rub up against your toes. Place a protective layer of moleskin or other cushioning over corn-prone
areas. Soften and peel existing corns with callus and corn plasters containing salicylic acid. If corns continue to be a source
of discomfort or pain, see a doctor about having bony defects
corrected.

Friction Blisters

I began to get lots of calls about blisters a few years ago. The
physical-fitness boom was still new then, and many of my patients decided to take up walking, jogging, weightlifting, and
other types of physical activity, without recognizing the impor-
tance of starting slowly and allowing tender skin to build up
protective calluses.

Blisters are caused by friction—rubbing. Even short periods
of chafing against uncallused skin can result in the sudden
eruption of a painful, fluid-filled blister. Blistering on feet is

usually a consequence of wearing ill-fitting shoes that rub against uncallused skin in the toe or heel area. A dramatic increase in activity—more walking or running than you're accustomed to—can result in blistering even when shoes fit comfortably.

The best thing to do for a blister is simply to keep skin in the area clean and dry and to cushion it, if necessary, with one of those doughnut-shaped pads. If the blister is on your foot, wear two layers of socks for workouts. (The inner sock should be made of a fabric that wicks moisture away from your skin— such as wool or polypropylene.) If a particular pair of shoes caused the problem, stop wearing them, of course. If they're too tight, you might want to see about having them stretched.

I wouldn't advise breaking a blister unless it is painful and located where continued rubbing will probably break it anyway. When that's the case, you might as well get relief by breaking and draining it yourself:

1. Wash the area with warm water and mild soap. Rinse and pat dry.

2. Sterilize a sharp needle by immersing it in boiling water for five minutes, or by holding it with tweezers over the flame of a gas stove for three minutes.

3. Use the needle to puncture the edge of the blister. Press gently with a sterile gauze pad until the fluid has drained out. Do not pull off or snip loose skin.

4. Apply an antibacterial ointment such as Bacitracin. Then cover the area with a sterile gauze pad held in place with adhesive tape.

Warts

Warts are caused by a virus that enters the skin, often through a tiny cut or abrasion, and infects the epidermis, the upper layer of skin cells. They often go away without treatment, according to a timetable all their own. No one, not even a dermatologist, can predict when a wart will disappear. With a single exception (more about that later), warts are rarely a health hazard, so unless they're painful or embarrassing, just waiting them out might be the best approach.

However, I know from talking with patients that there's a strong impulse to *do* something at the first sign of a wart. That usually means running out for some Compound W or one of the other over-the-counter remedies. These preparations sometimes work when applied daily for a period of weeks. If you decide to try one, be sure to use it exactly according to instructions on label or package insert.

If an over-the-counter product fails to deliver by the end of a month, and if you're in a hurry to get rid of the wart(s), see a doctor. Keep in mind, though, that even a highly skilled dermatologist employing the most sophisticated and advanced techniques won't guarantee immediate results. Warts are tricky. For instance, I recently treated a woman who had several small warts on her fingers. It looked as if we'd gotten rid of them right off the bat, but no such luck. They simply moved up to her hands, and those warts had to be treated as well.

There's no single best treatment for warts; there's a whole arsenal of different approaches—none of which work all the time for every type of wart. Sometimes it's necessary to try more than one.

For common warts, the rough-textured, well-defined, usually painless eruptions that turn up most often on hands, fingers, and knees, doctors often choose from among the following procedures:

• Cryosurgery, which freezes warts away by subjecting them for less than a minute to liquid nitrogen chilled to a temperature of $-195.5°C$. The super-cold causes tiny blisters to form and these in turn create a disturbance in virus-infected cells. When it works, it's a quick fix requiring no anesthesia. The procedure may need to be repeated for larger warts.

• Curettage, in which the entire wart is lifted out of the surrounding skin with a special instrument. The edges of the wart's "bed" are then scraped to remove remaining traces of virus-infected cells and prevent regrowth.

• Electrodessication, which, after the area is desensitized with an anesthetic, zaps warts with a high-frequency electrical current delivered by a needle. Within a few hours after the procedure, a crust or scab usually forms. When it drops off, the wart goes along with it. We hope.

• Chemosurgery, in which chemicals such as trichloracetic acid, salicylic acid, phenol, and/or silver nitrate—or a phenol-nitric-salicylic acid paste—are topically applied. The chemicals induce peeling and/or crusting which dislodge the growth. If all goes well.

• Carbon dioxide laser surgery, which uses a focused beam of high-intensity light to "vaporize" the wart, leaving the area flatter and smoother. (To inhibit regrowth and the development of new warts near the site, I sometimes use the laser, set at a lower intensity, to "brush" over areas adjacent to the wart under treatment.)

For small, scattered facial warts, tretinoin (Retin-A), which peels off upper skin cell layers, is sometimes successful.

Warts occurring near or under fingernails are called *periungual warts*. People who bite or pick at their fingernails and cuticles are somewhat more likely to be infected periungually. The virus responsible for these warts can be picked up from manicure implements used by others afflicted with the growths—a good reason not to borrow manicure equipment and to make sure that tools and equipment used in salons are disinfected after each use. Periungual warts can be painful and will cost a fingernail if they grow in the nail bed under a nail. They're also among the most difficult to treat.

In the last couple of years, bleomycin, a cancer drug, has been used with some success on particularly resistant periungual warts. The procedure involves injecting a dilute solution of the drug directly into the growth. It can be painful and may need to be repeated at two- or three-week intervals. Bleomycin is considered a last resort treatment to be used only on stubborn warts that have been present for six months or more. But when all else fails, it does offer some hope of improvement for intractable growths.

A *plantar wart*, so-called because it occurs on the plantar or bottom surface of the foot, is another treatment-resistant growth. One way to minimize your chances of getting a plantar wart is to keep your shoes on when you're away from home. The virus causing it is most likely to be picked up at public swimming pools, gyms, hotel bathrooms, and in other places where people tend to go barefoot.

A plantar wart typically makes its initial appearance as a small dot on the sole of the foot. Picking or poking at it with fingernails or a sharp instrument can cause it to grow bigger. (I've seen some that covered most of the weight-bearing surface of the foot. Warts that large, especially if they are also deep-rooted, can make walking extremely uncomfortable.)

Formalin, chemically related to formaldehyde, is often the treatment of choice for plantar warts. After application of the chemical, the growth is covered with tape containing salicylic acid, which helps the formalin penetrate. When the tape is removed, several layers of dead skin cells, including part of the wart, come off along with it. The procedure may need to be repeated several times. More of the wart is removed each time the tape is taken off, and what's left becomes drier and begins to scale. Depending on the size of the growth, it can take anywhere from a few days to several weeks to get rid of it.

Genital warts, also known as *venereal warts*, occurring in the ano-genital area, are moist, pink or gray, and tend to resemble a cauliflower in shape and texture (but not in size; the warts are much smaller). Whether or not these warts cause pain or discomfort, they should be looked at by a doctor. *Buschke-Lowenstein giant condyloma*, a type of genital wart found most frequently in people over the age of forty, is the only wart that, if left untreated, can turn cancerous.

Moles

Though moles are technically tumors of the skin, the vast majority of them are benign—simply clusters of pigmented cells ranging in color from an almost-invisible flesh tone to bluish-black. Some are flat and smooth; some are raised and hairy; some have a grainy texture similar to fine sandpaper. Most often they appear in the first decade or so of life, though some form in middle age. Congenital moles, the ones you were born with, are more likely to turn cancerous than others, especially if they are large, flat, dark-colored, and covered with coarse hair. Many dermatologists urge removal of moles fitting this description at an early age.

However, if you notice *any* change in the size, shape, color, or texture of *any* mole, or if a mole becomes sensitive, painful, or itchy, or begins to bleed or ooze, see a doctor immediately. Any of these changes could be a sign of malignancy.

There's a terrific quick remedy for almost any mole that bothers you for cosmetic reasons: Hide it with one of the excellent products developed to tone out pigmentation irregularities. Dermablend Cover Creme is probably best known, but there are several others. Used according to manufacturer's instructions, they do a great job and I heartily recommend them.

Removal of moles you don't like the looks of can be a good idea, especially if your surgeon is skilled in working within natural skin folds and is deft in suturing. But every dermatologist recognizes that in a small percentage of cases of purely elective surgery, done for cosmetic reasons only, it makes sense to leave well enough alone. Unfortunately, it's not always easy to convince the patient.

A couple of years ago a woman came in to my office and wanted to have every mole on her body removed. There must have been about a hundred of them, but none were especially conspicuous and most were very small and light brown. I told her to show me the three or four moles she was most eager to be rid of, and I'd decide if—based on their location—there was a good chance of removing them without visible scarring. We proceeded on that basis; I excised the moles; and she healed without scarring, just as I'd expected. Apparently, she wasn't happy with my cautious approach. Months went by and I didn't see her again until she came to the office about a rash. "I guess you decided to keep those moles," I remarked. "I wish I had," she responded. She'd been living overseas. A European surgeon had granted her wish and removed most of the moles, and she was left with a scattering of small scars to remember them by. It came down to trading one kind of minor flaw for another.

When is it better to leave well enough alone? Only your doctor can make a final determination, of course. I take into consideration the location of the mole—some areas heal better than others—and, if scarring is a possibility, whether it can be hidden in an expression line or skin fold. I also consider pigmentation. Individuals with black, brown, or Mediterranean skin tend to scar more easily than lighter, blue-eyed people.

Mole removal for health or beauty reasons is relatively quick and simple—an example of what I call "lunch-hour surgery," because the patient is usually in and out of the doctor's office in that amount of time. And believe it or not, the procedures are almost always painless.

In "shaving," the surface of the mole is sliced off with a scalpel, then the skin surface is smoothed with an electric needle. In surgical excision, the mole is removed with a scalpel and if necessary the area is closed with sutures. In electrocauterization, the mole is seared off by means of an electric hot-wire tool. I do not use this last method, since it destroys the mole, leaving nothing for a biopsy.

"Barnacles" (*Seborrheic Keratoses*)

They're not really barnacles, of course, but that's what these bumpy brownish or yellowish, often scaly growths that appear to be stuck onto the skin look like to some of my patients. (Though one woman said they reminded her of candle wax.)

Harmless but decidedly unattractive, they're sometimes mistaken for warts.

Luckily, they're a lot easier to get rid of than warts. Most often, one of the lunch-hour surgical techniques described in the section on moles is all it takes. Seborrheic keratoses can also be frozen with liquid nitrogen or scraped off with an instrument called a curette.

Cherry Angiomas

Actually clusters of overgrown capillaries, these small, round, raised growths are dark red—thus the name. I usually remove them by electrosurgery or with a laser; in many cases there is not even a suggestion that a procedure was performed.

Skin Tags

Loose, flesh-colored flaps of skin that are usually just a little bigger than the head of a pin, skin tags occur most frequently on the neck and near the armpits or groin. I also see a lot of them around the eyes. They're among the simplest skin irregularities to remove. Getting rid of them is so simple in fact that some of my patients who had them for years say they could "kick themselves" for not having them taken care of earlier. In electrodesiccation, tags are blitzed with a weak current delivered through an electric needle. Easier still, tags can be snipped off with surgical scissors. Aftercare is usually just a matter of gently washing the area with mild soap and water. (I advise patients who've had tags removed from near their eyes not to wear eye makeup for a while.)

Birthmarks

Port wine stains are the most common "vascular" birthmarks, or *hemangiomas*, which are composed primarily of enlarged

blood vessels. Often, they're very pale and almost impercepti-
ble in infancy. However, in later years, as more blood vessels
develop, they can turn red or purplish, thicken, and take on a
roughened, pebbly texture. Though they're harmless, they can
be a source of great emotional discomfort, especially when they
are located in areas not ordinarily covered by clothing.

Special coverup makeup, such as that made by Dermablend,
can block out port wine stains. The makeup is available at department stores and most well-stocked pharmacies and comes
with complete, easy-to-read instructions, including guidelines
for how to achieve subtle, natural-looking results.

The new pulse laser is the most effective means of removing
port wine stains and other hemangiomas. In this procedure a
focused beam of yellow light is delivered in short pulses at very
high repetition rates, making it appear continuous to the naked eye. Yellow light is also ideal for other blood vessel abnormalities such as spider veins, cherry angiomas, and "broken
blood vessels" associated with acne rosacea. Since there are
different types of lasers, the dermatologist may have to experiment with several in varying intensities to see which is most
effective. (The laser works by stimulating new collagen formation in the area. The collagen in turn surrounds dilated blood
vessels, constricting them enough to return them to normal or
almost normal size.) A scab forms over the laser-treated areas,
and when it falls off, the skin underneath is flatter and lighter
in color. Repeated treatments usually result in further lightening and flattening of the birthmark.

Stretch Marks

As the name suggests, these lines and grooves appearing on
breasts, abdomen, hips, buttocks, thighs, and sometimes on upper arms and back, are caused by prolonged, drastic stretching
of the skin. The marks are actually "fractures" of the skin, which
occur within the dermis. These develop when elastin and col-

lagen fibers are pulled to the point where resiliency and tone—the ability to snap back, like a rubber band—are affected.

If you've got stretch marks, you're in excellent company. The great majority of pregnant women (about 90 percent) develop them as their breasts enlarge and their abdomens distend to accommodate the growth of the unborn baby. Marks show up, too, on many preteens and teenagers during the fleshing-out period of the adolescent growth spurt. Some bodybuilders are afflicted when muscle tissue increases enough to place abnormal strain on the overlying skin. In fact, anyone who for any reason experiences a rapid, dramatic gain in weight or bulk is a candidate for stretch marks. Once there, the marks are permanent.

Yes, permanent. So far, there's not a thing you can do to get rid of them short of removing the affected skin. However, the reddish or purplish color of "new" stretch marks gradually fades to a shade somewhat lighter than surrounding skin, sometimes becoming all but invisible.

Every year around the time my patients begin to think about sun, sand, and bathing suits, I'm bombarded with requests for something—anything—to get rid of stretch marks. My standard response is, "forget about the marks." Nine times out of ten, the only person who notices them is the one who has them. If that advice isn't good enough, though, I suggest using a cosmetic camouflage, such as Dermablend Cover Creme. It's opaque enough to hide stretch marks, comes in a range of shades to blend in with any skin color, is easy to apply, and once on, it's waterproof.

Other options are more drastic. For example, sections of stretch-marked skin might be removed in the course of surgical procedures performed to remove excess abdominal skin.

Dermabrasion is another approach, though I wouldn't recommend it because of the possibility of scarring.

Emolliant, lubricating products containing lanolin, vitamin E, petrolatum, and cocoa butter will not help reduce stretch marks!

How to Prevent Stretch Marks

Since they're impossible to remove without resorting to surgery, it makes sense to try to avoid getting stretch marks in the first place. Here are my suggestions:

• Try to maintain your weight at or near what's considered ideal for your height and bone structure. (If you're in doubt about your best weight, check out the ubiquitous height/weight charts of Metropolitan Life Insurance Company. Almost every diet book has them.) Weight gain, especially rapid weight gain, puts enormous stress on the skin, so avoid yo-yoing—gaining, losing, gaining, and so on.
• Of course, follow your obstetrician's dietary guidelines when you are pregnant. Gaining a certain number of pounds (your physician will tell you approximately how many) is normal and healthy for you and your baby-to-be. But don't exceed your doctor's recommendations. Pregnancy is prime-time for stretch marks.
• Don't go on crash weight-lifting or body-building programs designed to pump up your muscles unless you are willing to accept stretch marks as a possible consequence.

Incidentally, aerobic activities—walking, swimming, bicycling, aerobic dancing, et cetera—are unlikely to cause stretch marks. These exercises, which promote cardiovascular fitness, also enhance muscle tone, but for women do not usually result in the kind of overdevelopment that places a strain on skin.

Cellulite

"Dimpled" skin on thighs, hips, rear, and in some cases upper arms is a problem, I suppose. I know that many, many women are very concerned about it. But it's been oversold as an abnormality. The truth is, "cellulite" is a normal consequence of being a woman. The orange-rind appearance of cellulite is due to the presence of fat cells clustered in clumps close to the surface of the skin. Over years, as skin thins, loses tone—and especially if there is weight gain—fat-cell clusters may become more visible. Every once in a while an exasperated female patient will point to her overweight husband and ask, "Why doesn't *he* have cellulite?" The answer has to do with the fact that most men have a different pattern of fat distribution, and thicker skin, than most women.

I'm not suggesting that you learn to love your cellulite and leave it at that. Only that it's not a disease, and that in fact, it exists to some degree in almost all women (female athletes seem to be the exception), and especially in older women whose skin has begun to thin. Of course, the more subcutaneous fat there is, the more evident cellulite will be.

My aim in writing this book has been to give you the information you need to solve your own beauty problems quickly and easily, but there's no quick and easy cure for this nondisease. Not that you can't make improvements. A good, sensible diet, if you are overweight, coupled with an exercise program preferably based on aerobic activities, should result in less cellulite simply because diet and exercise will reduce the amount of fat on your body.

As for those scrapers, mitts, and other devices touted as cellulite "cures," I've seen no evidence to indicate that any of them do any good. Not surprising, since manipulating the surface of the skin does not affect the amount and distribution of the fat underneath. Plastic sweatpants, injections, pills, and expensive treatments that involve wrapping the problem areas in fabric soaked with special "anticellulite" solutions are equally ineffective. Save your money.

Liposuction (also called *suction lipectomy*), in which pockets of fat are vacuumed away by means of a blunt, tubelike instrument inserted under the skin, may be an option if you are relatively slim but have localized, diet- and exercise-resistant fat pockets on hips, rear, thighs, and so on. However, the procedure is not for everyone and can result in rippled skin in the areas from which fat was removed—an outcome potentially as unaesthetic as the original problem.

"Road Map" Thighs

When one of my patients complained that her legs looked like road maps, I knew what she meant even before I took a look. She had what are often called *spider veins*. These are wiggly or threadlike bluish or red lines, sometimes connected in a sunburst pattern resembling a spider. Not to be confused with the much larger varicose veins, spider veins are small blood vessels that have become enlarged. Because they carry more blood than normal-size vessels, they are visible through the skin.

Spider veins can be a beauty problem when they are numerous. The quickest, easiest solution is simply to cover them up with an opaque camouflage cream, such as Dermablend.

When and if you decide to do something more about spider veins, talk with a dermatologist. Although blood does flow through these veins (spider veins aren't "broken," as many people assume) they are not essential to good circulation and often can be eradicated. Many doctors prefer sclerotherapy to treat spider veins on legs. This procedure involves injection of a special solution that irritates the walls of the vessel. A tiny blood clot forms and the walls begin to disintegrate; blood and the disintegrated vessel are gradually absorbed by the body and disappear. There may be a minor discomfort, redness, and swelling in the area for a day or so. Some spider veins need to be treated two or three times over a period of weeks or months. Larger ones might return—though often the "reappearance" of an old one is really a new one near the old site. Other treatments for spider veins are laser surgery and electrosurgery (also called electrodesiccation), performed with current delivered by a very fine needle. However, I avoid using these methods because of the possibility of scarring.

Electrosurgery is often the preferred treatment for enlarged veins on the face, which tend to be more "resistant" to sclerotherapy. (Scarring is less likely here because facial skin can be treated with current of a lower intensity.) The new pulse laser is another excellent method for eliminating facial veins.

Preventing Road Map Thighs

Heredity seems to play a role in who will have spider veins and when. So does estrogen—the normal amount you have as a woman and the kind you get as an ingredient in birth control pills or in estrogen replacement therapy. There isn't much you can do about either, but you can control some of the other factors thought to make spider veins more likely.

•Avoid prolonged exposure to intense sun. (Here is still another reason to wear a sunscreen on the face and body when you go outdoors.)

• Limit your intake of alcohol and caffeine, both of which tend to dilate blood vessels.

• Don't overmanipulate your skin. Rough massage, excessive friction, or pummeling during exercise or other activities can damage blood vessels close to the surface of the skin, and may increase the likelihood of spider veins.

Hair You Don't Want

There are a number of options for dealing with excess hair, but none of them are all-purpose. The guidelines below will tell you which hair-removal methods are most appropriate for use on various parts of the body and how to achieve the best results.

Shaving

Good for getting rid of hair under arms and on legs from the knees down.

Pros. Shaving is cheap; it's fast; all you need is a razor, soap, and water; and you can do it almost anywhere, anytime—even daily if hair is dark and regrowth is rapid and conspicuous.

Cons. Since shaved hair is lopped off at the surface of the skin—instead of being pulled out by the roots or dissolved slightly below the surface, as in some other methods—regrowth may be noticeable within a day or so and often feels stubbly or prickly. (Shaving, of course, does not cause hair to become thicker or coarser, but because shaved hair is "blunt cut" instead of "tapered," it feels stiff and bristly as it grows in.) Skin can be nicked or cut if the razor is not used with care.

How to Get a Quick, Close Shave

• Don't shave first thing in the morning when fluids that accumulate overnight can make body skin somewhat puffy. You'll get a closer shave later on when fluids have dispersed. For the same reason, don't shave before or during a long soak in the tub when skin may be "waterlogged." Shaving after a brief shower is okay, though it makes more sense to me to shave first and shower or bathe later to wash away stray hairs. Do not shave right before swimming in salt water or a chlorinated pool. Even careful shaving can irritate skin; salt or chlorine will add to your discomfort.

• A sharp blade is a must. I like disposable razors which can be used two or three times and then tossed. Disposable or not, a blade is too dull to give a close shave if it pulls or drags as you stroke it across your skin.

• Wash the area to be shaved with soap and water as hot as you can comfortably tolerate. Do not dry. Moisture left on for a minute or so will soften hairs and help you get a cleaner shave. If your skin is very easily irritated, apply a moisturizing lotion or light oil, such as baby oil, instead of washing.

• Work soap into a rich lather and smooth onto areas to be shaved. Or use a shaving cream or gel; these products were developed to reduce friction between skin and blade, and most are less drying than soap.

• Shave *against* hair growth. Stroke lightly, using as little pressure as possible. Don't scrape.

• Don't shave vertically along shinbones—the long bones between knees and ankles. In this area, shaving on the diagonal tends to result in fewer nicks and cuts.

• To prevent a buildup of shaved hairs from interfering with clean shaving, rinse the razor frequently as you work.

• Instead of using an astringent, toner, or after-shave product containing alcohol, which can sting and increase irritation, soothe just-shaved areas with talc or a moisturizer.

• Wait at least an hour after shaving, longer if possible, before applying deodorant or antiperspirant. Most contain ingredients that sting and which may increase irritation after shaving.

Shaving and Ingrown Hairs

Many of the problems associated with shaving, including the stinging and bumpy redness many women experience afterward, can be avoided by following the guidelines above. These same suggestions should also reduce the incidence of ingrown hairs—hair tips that have curled under and grow back into the skin. However, if ingrowth continues, as it sometimes does in curly haired women and men, consider switching to an electric shaver. Scouring the area gently with a loofah or polyester facial sponge between shavings can help too. (Mild abrasion will remove some of the upper layers of dead skin cells where hair that curls back on itself can get trapped.)

Waxing

Appropriate for large areas, including legs, arms, the bikini area, and for removing facial hair (down on upper lips and cheeks), the stripe of hair running from navel to pubic area, and the fuzz on toes.

Pros. In waxing, hair is pulled from the follicles, well below the surface of the skin, so results are smoother and longer lasting than in shaving. New hair tends to grow in naturally, with tapered tips, so regrowth isn't bristly. Slight damage to the follicle as hair is yanked out may cause it to produce softer, finer hair with successive waxings.

Cons. Do-it-yourself waxing can be uncomfortable, even painful, unless you have the technique down pat. Salon waxing, done by an experienced pro, is less uncomfortable, but more expensive. Stripping off any type of wax may irritate delicate, sensitive skin. Finally, if it's important that you be hair-free at all times, waxing may not be a good option, since you must wait until regrowth is at least one-quarter inch long before rewaxing.

Tips for Do-It-Yourself Hot Waxing

This method of hair removal involves melting wax, or a waxlike material, until it is spreadable and applying it evenly. Individual hairs are caught in the wax as it hardens and are pulled out when the wax is stripped off.

• Have the job done at a salon the first time. Watching a professional at work, and asking questions about the procedure, will give you a better understanding of how to do it yourself.
• Inspect areas to be waxed to make sure there are no open cuts, abrasions, redness, or irritation. Dust lightly with baby powder or talc before applying wax.
• Test the temperature of melted wax by placing a very small amount on a relatively hair-free area such as the inside of your arm. It should be the consistency of toothpaste—not runny—and warm enough to spread, *but not hot.* Be aware that very hot wax can cause a severe burn since it cannot easily be removed before it has cooled enough to become slightly hard.
• When you are absolutely sure wax is cool enough not to burn, apply a smooth, even coating. Detour around any moles, birthmarks, or warts. (Protect these areas with a film of petroleum jelly.) The best way to apply wax is to hold skin taut with one hand and with the other spread wax in the direction of hair growth. (If your kit came with a cloth to facilitate wax removal, now is the time to press the cloth gently onto the wax.)

• Remove wax when it is still warm, but no longer sticky. If you wait until it cools, it may crack as you try to get a grip on it. Grasp an end in one hand (or, if you have applied a cloth, take one end of it in your hand), hold skin taut with the other, and pull it off against the direction of the hair growth in one quick, decisive motion. To rid your skin of stray bits and pieces of wax, press down on them with a strip of still-warm, freshly removed wax. (Heat from the wax will soften the flecks, and they'll come off with the strip.) Or apply baby oil and rub or pick flecks off with your fingers.

• Soothe just-waxed skin by covering with a clean cloth dipped in icy-cold water and wrung out. Press it down firmly on areas that sting. Blot dry and apply a moisturizing lotion.

Cold Waxing

In this system of hair removal, wax or a waxlike substance is bonded onto strips of paper or fabric. The waxy side is pressed on skin to be treated, then the strip is pulled off.

The cold wax strips I've seen seem to work best on small areas where hair is fine or downy and not very thick, such as on upper lip, cheeks, and in some women the line of hair from navel to pubic area. Coarser hair on calves, under arms, and in the bikini area can be removed more efficiently by other means.

Cream Depilatories

These creams work chemically, by dissolving hair to the point where it can be wiped away. They can be used to get rid of unwanted hair almost anywhere. The exceptions are strays around nipples and near organs that might be harmed by accidental contact with the products. (For example, because they're so near eyes, you should not use a depilatory to remove eyebrow strays.)

Pros. Smooth-on, roll-on, and foam-on depilatories are easy to use, inexpensive, and work fairly quickly (hair is dissolved in five to fifteen minutes, depending on amount and texture). Hair is dissolved at or just below the surface of the skin; results are somewhat longer-lasting than those obtained in shaving, and regrowth is less bristly.

Cons. Chemical ingredients in depilatories are related to those used in permanent wave solutions and can irritate sensitive skin. (Most skin is not adversely affected when products are properly used, according to instructions on the label.) There's a certain amount of mess involved, even with roll-on application. And though the chemical odor—something like that of a perm solution—is masked with fragrance, it's still there.

How to Get Better Results with a Cream Depilatory

• As with any product, use it according to the manufacturer's instructions. Smooth it on so that it completely covers all hair to be removed. It's important not to allow a depilatory to remain on skin longer than the recommended time. If a time range for coarse hair is given—say, ten to fifteen minutes—at the end of ten minutes wipe a small area with a dampened cloth. If hair comes off easily, there's no need to wait any longer; go ahead and wipe all treated areas. Otherwise, wait a minute or two and try again. If hair can't be wiped away at the end of the recommended time, it's highly resistant to chemical depilation. Rather than leave the product on longer and risk irritation, wipe it off and rinse away remaining traces. You'll have to consider other methods of hair removal.
• To reduce any redness or stinging after using a depilatory, dip a clean cloth in very cold water, wring it out, and press gently on treated areas.
• Wait several hours or overnight before applying deodorant

to depilated underarms and before using a toner, freshener, or other product containing alcohol on areas from which facial hair has been removed.

Tweezing

Removing individual hairs with tweezers is the method of choice for neatening eyebrows and getting rid of strays else-where on the body. The exceptions are hairs growing from moles and in the nose and ears. These should be clipped with scissors.

Pros. Tweezing is cheap, though an initial investment in good tweezers with tips that meet exactly is a must. It's neat, and it's precise, allowing you to remove one hair at a time. Since hair is pulled out from below the surface, regrowth isn't usually apparent for several weeks.

Cons. Tweezing is impractical for mass removal of hairs from large areas. Another drawback for many women is the sting. And like some other methods of hair removal, tweezing can result in ingrown hairs, especially in curly haired individuals.

For advice on how to tweeze safely and as painlessly as possible, see the section on eyebrows, beginning on page 59 in Chapter 3.

Epilady and Similar Devices

This plug-in beauty appliance resembles an electric razor in size and shape but functions more like automated tweezers. The machine, with its rotating coil head that grasps and pulls out hairs from below the surface, works best on large areas, such as forearms and legs.

Pros. The appliance is easy to use, won't nick or scrape, and there's no mess. Because hair is plucked out of the follicle, results are long lasting and regrowth tends to be finer, softer, and less abundant, as in waxing. Once you get the hang of using the device, hair removal is quick—it should take about ten minutes to do both legs.

Cons. Because many hairs are pulled out at once, some stinging is to be expected, at least the first few times the machine is used. I've talked to patients who tell me they've become so accustomed to the stinging, it no longer bothers them. But others, often women with very coarse hair, have said that because of discomfort, they had to give up on this procedure and go back to more traditional methods of hair removal. Epilady is most effective when hair is at least one-quarter inch long, so there can be an awkward growing-out period between sessions.

Everything you need to know to achieve optimal results is included in the instructions that come with the appliance.

Electrolysis

The only permanent method for getting rid of unwanted hair, electrolysis is done with a very fine needle, or probe, which is inserted into individual hair follicles and destroys them with heat, chemicals, or a combination of the two. In theory, hair can be removed from any area by means of electrolysis, but the procedure is most often used to clean up small areas, such as upper lip, cheeks, chin, and, less often, the bikini area.

Pros. Though it may take two or three sessions to destroy some follicles, permanent removal of embarrassing hair on cheeks or chin is a definite plus.

Cons. The procedure can be painful and sometimes leaves small scars. The potential for pain and scarring has been reduced by the development of an insulated probe (IB probe), which ensures that the current is discharged only when it makes contact with tissue surrounding the root of the hair. Nevertheless, women who are left with a dark spot or discoloration after a pimple heals may experience similar pigment changes in areas treated by electrolyis. (Black and olive-skinned women are most at risk for such changes.) Since follicles must be destroyed one by one, and any single follicle might need to be zapped more than once, permanent hair removal by this method can take weeks or months, depending on the size of the area. Even when results appear to be permanent, a few follow-up treatments may be necessary to keep treated areas completely hair-free. At $20 to $50 or more per session, electrolysis isn't cheap.

Tips for Getting Better Results with Electrolysis

• Choose an electrologist with care. Personal recommendations from friends or acquaintances can steer you in the right direction. But even a glowing report from someone you know should not outweigh lack of professional accreditation from the American Electrology Association. For the names of professionals working in your area, call the Association (201/466-1975) or ask your dermatologist for a referral.

• Schedule appointments so that you do not undergo treatment on the two or three days before and after the start of a menstrual period. Fluid rentention at those times can make your skin puffier, which may in turn affect results. (Some women are more sensitive to pain right before and after the onset of a period.)

• Use calamine lotion to soothe freshly treated skin. If electrolysis was performed on your face, don't wear makeup for several hours or until the next day.

• Consider whether you are a good candidate for this method of hair removal before you proceed with it. For example, I urge my patients who are diabetics not to undergo electrolysis, since they are more susceptible to infection and its consequences than others. I do not recommend electrolysis for my black patients since they are more at risk for heavy scarring and skin color changes. Men and women who wear cardiac pacemakers should not have electrolysis because the pacemaker might be affected by electrical current delivered by the probe. Young teens may develop more hair as they mature and should put off treatment until at least the age of seventeen.

Bleaching

If hair is dark but not profuse, lightening it a few shades to make it less conspicuous is often a good solution, especially for small areas, such as the upper lip, cheeks, chin, and for some women, their forearms.

Pros. Stubbly regrowth is never a problem since hair is not removed. Depending on the rate at which old hairs are shed and new hairs take their place, results can last as long as four weeks, and the darkening is gradual. Do-it-yourself bleaching is easy and relatively inexpensive. (Products designed to bleach facial and body hair are available at department stores and well-stocked drugstores. Do not use hair-color products on your face or body.)

Cons. Chemicals in the bleach can irritate sensitive skin—or *any* skin if the bleach is left on too long. Very dark hair may turn an unattractive and unnatural-looking orange shade.

Guidelines for Better Bleaching

• Read and follow carefully all instructions printed on the package insert. Don't neglect to do a patch test to determine your sensitivity to the product if that is recommended by the manufacturer.

• To make sure you get the right degree of lightening, without conspicuous brassiness, test-bleach a small area on your arm before treating facial hair. Apply the bleach, wait five to seven minutes, then check the color. If it's too dark, too yellow, or too orange, leave it on for another few minutes. Do not exceed the time limit suggested in the package insert. Bleaching is not for you if your hair does not lighten up enough within the allotted time.

• After bleaching, apply a moisturizer to soften and soothe.

• Though instructions that come with some bleaches give directions for lightening eyebrows, I don't recommend this as a do-it-yourself procedure. Chemicals strong enough to change hair color are too strong for anyone but a skilled professional to use so close to your eyes. If you think your eyebrows are too dark, have them lightened by a professional at a good salon.

Dos and Don'ts for Removing Hair in "Ticklish Places"

Nose Hair

Longish hairs sprouting from within the nostrils are a cause of embarrassment for some. Occasionally, a patient will ask about electrolysis as a way to permanently remove these hairs. I don't recommend it. Skin inside the nose is very sensitive to pain. Because of this, a weaker current is often used to eradicate hair in the area. However, because the current is weaker, it may take several sessions to destroy the follicles.

Less painful and less expensive is to use small, sharp scissors to clip hair near the openings of the nostrils. Do not try to snip hairs farther inside the nose. Because you can't see what you're doing, there's a greater risk of cutting yourself.

Bikini Line Hair

Shaving leaves the area feeling itchy and irritated, and the rapid, stubbly regrowth is almost as unattractive in a revealing swimsuit as longer hairs. Epilady is not recommended for the bikini area. Bleaching doesn't really solve the problem. And tweezing is much too painful and tedious. That leaves waxing and depilation. Waxing involves some discomfort, but results will last longer and regrowth should be finer. (Cold wax may not be up to the job if hair is very coarse and thick.) Depilation doesn't hurt, but you'll have to be careful not to allow the product to come into contact with the genitals.

Whichever method you choose, the job will be easier and results neater if you first slip into an old pair of bikini underpants. They'll protect and also provide convenient guidelines for applying the wax or depilatory.

Hair on Breasts and Nipples

A few stray hairs on the breast are usual, and even a light down is normal. With the exception of Epilady, you can use any of the methods described in this section to remove hair surrounding nipples. However, hair on breasts should not be removed while you are pregnant or breastfeeding; at these times, breast skin is more sensitive than usual. It's also important to avoid contact with nipples, moles, birthmarks, and irritated areas.

Hair growing from nipples is another matter. Tweezing and clipping are the only safe ways to remove it. Use sterilized tweezers and follow up with a dab of alcohol. If tweezing hurts too much, clip carefully with a pair of small, sharp scissors. Hold breast skin taut with one hand to elevate the base of the hair. Snip with the other hand, being careful not to clip too close to skin.

When Excess Hair Could Signal Trouble

If you've always been hairier than you'd like, chances are the condition is inherited and normal for you. But any sudden increase in hair on your chest, breasts, back, or face could indicate a hormone imbalance or other problem. Check it out with a doctor.

Problem Perspiration

Except for a very few unfortunate individuals afflicted with congenital *anhidrotic ectodermal defect* (total or near-total absence of sweat glands), everyone perspires all the time. Sweat glands produce more perspiration in warm weather and during exercise, and that is as it should be; the moisture cools as it evaporates, enabling the body to tolerate warm environments and brisk activity without overheating. But profuse perspiration that is not related to heat or activity can be a problem. Perpetual dampness under arms, on palms, and elsewhere may be a response to anxiety or stress, or it could be genetic in origin. Almost always, there's a way to control it.

Stay-Dry Guidelines for Underarms

• First, take a look at the product you've been using under your arms. If it's a deodorant, it's meant to control or prevent unpleasant odor. It was not formulated to combat sweating. Only antiperspirants and antiperspirant/deodorants will do that. The solution to your problem might be as simple as switching from a deodorant to an antiperspirant/deodorant.

• Even an antiperspirant won't control excessive sweating if you don't give it a chance. The active ingredient in many antiperspirants is an aluminum salt, often aluminum chloride—though products containing aluminum chlorhydrate or zirconium aluminum tend to be even better at controlling perspiration. All these aluminum salts work by forming gelatinous "plugs" which partially block sweat ducts and prevent perspiration from reaching the surface. It takes five to ten days of regular use of an antiperspirant for plugs to form and everyday application thereafter to keep them in pace. A swipe at your underarms every few days just won't do it.

• Be aware that different formulations have varying degrees of effectiveness. As a general rule, aerosol products are less efficient than solid, stick-form antiperspirants, while roll-ons offer the best protection of all. Before applying a roll-on, shake it up; some of the active ingredients can settle to the bottom of the container.

• Because moisture dilutes the ingredients and encourages dissolution of those little plugs, don't apply your antiperspirant immediately after shower or bath. Instead, pat underarms good and dry after bathing and wait several minutes. Better yet, use an antiperspirant right before bed so that it can act on pore openings overnight without interference from moisture.

• Underarm hair, when it's allowed to grow too long, provides an ideal environment for odor-causing bacteria. Daily hair removal isn't necessary and could lead to irritation. Once a week should be enough.

• Clothing made of natural fibers that absorb moisture—cotton, wool, silk, linen—is preferable to those made of synthetics (polyesters, acrylics, nylon, etc.), which are nonabsorbent, tend to trap moisture (perspiration), and prevent evaporation.

If the suggestions above aren't enough to keep you drier, see a dermatologist. He or she can prescribe a stronger antiperspirant, such as Drysol, or, in extreme cases, a special electronic device made by the Drionic Company in California. The unit is applied to underarms (there are other units for hands and feet) for a few minutes every day until sweat glands are deactivated.

Excessive sweating, or *hyperhidrosis*, is not that unusual. In many people it's genetic. For others, the condition may be linked to diabetes, thyroid abnormalities, certain neurological disorders, or obesity. Treatment of the underlying problem sometimes helps control sweating as well.

Clammy Hands

Perspiration problems aren't limited to underarms. Some of my patients are cool as the proverbial cucumber, except for their hands. When the condition isn't too severe, this simple do-it-yourself remedy can be very helpful:

1. Wash your hands, rinse with cool water, and pat thoroughly dry.

2. Apply antiperspirant to palms only.

3. Reapply antiperspirant every time you wash your hands, and in between times, if necessary.

You might also want to keep a small bottle of astringent, witch hazel, or light cologne in your handbag. When it's not convenient to wash your hands, a few drops of any of these, rubbed into palms and blotted with a tissue, will encourage moisture evaporation and help keep your hands drier.

Dermatologists can prescribe stronger measures if you need them. But we can't come looking for you. Carole, a young woman whose hands perspired so profusely she wouldn't date, wouldn't dance, wouldn't shake hands—and in fact avoided almost all situations in which she might have to touch another person—waited years before seeing a doctor, partly because she was so self-conscious about the condition she could hardly bring herself to talk about it. She was relieved when I told her she wasn't the only person in the world with sweaty hands and astonished when the antiperspirant prescribed for her actually worked. She only regretted not coming for help sooner.

Sweaty Feet

When feet perspire excessively, odor is almost always a problem too. Here's a plan of attack for countering this double trouble.

1. Bathe or shower with a deodorant soap, such as Dial, paying special attention to your feet.

2. Pat feet completely dry, making sure to blot up all moisture between toes. Wait a few minutes, then apply an antiperspirant to the soles of your feet and between your toes.

3. Before getting into stockings, dust your feet with baking soda or a commercial deodorant foot powder.

4. At bedtime, soak your feet for several minutes in Burow's

Solution, available at drugstores. Dry thoroughly and reapply antiperspirant.

Place odor-absorbent cushioning in your shoes. Whenever possible, change to fresh stockings and shoes during the day. Because they're porous and allow feet to "breathe," leather shoes are a better choice than footwear of synthetic leather, plastic, or rubber. Once again, if you need more help, see a doctor. A prescription antiperspirant, sweat-control unit, or other measures should bring significant improvement.

9

Stop-the-Clock Techniques for a Younger Look

Skin around the eyes slackens, creating puffiness above and below. Frown lines etch themselves in the forehead. Corners of the mouth droop and deep folds appear from nose to mouth. The chin and jawline lose their clean, taut look and the neck turns crepey. There's a decrease in skin elasticity; it becomes looser and literally too big to fit neatly over underlying muscle and bone. Eventually it hangs like an oversize garment, in a series of sags and folds.

What's the timetable for all this? It depends—on the genes passed on to you, on the way you've chosen to live your life, on all the things you've done or haven't done to and for your skin over the years. But no matter when signs of aging begin to appear, it's always too soon.

You can't turn back the clock. Aging is inevitable. But there are ways to camouflage some of the visible signs of getting older and things you can do to minimize and even erase other signs. And most important, there are steps you can take to slow the process.

The Truth About Commercial "Anti-Agers"

No discussion about ways to counter skin aging should begin without first assessing some of those "fountain-of-youth" products developed to help make their users look younger. Virtually every company in the beauty business has a line of "anti-agers." My patients are always asking, "Can this cream (or lotion or gel or serum) really take years off my face?" I tell them what I'm going to tell you.

If you've been neglecting your skin for years, the new products may make you look better. Possibly even a lot better.

But if you've been taking good care of your skin all along— protecting it from the sun, treating it properly according to type, eating a healthy, well-balanced diet, exercising moderately, getting enough sleep, avoiding tobacco and drugs, and not overindulging in alcohol—chances are, anti-aging products won't make a significant difference.

Many of the new products are moisturizers, souped up with high-tech ingredients and/or old-standard substances (such as herbs and other botanicals, vitamins, thymus gland extracts, and placental compounds) presented in new guises. Often, these super-moisturizers come in innovative formats, such as ampoules and microcapsules. The new delivery systems were created to help ingredients penetrate better and more deeply into the skin. Nevertheless, they function in pretty much the same way as ordinary moisturizers: By supplying and binding moisture to cells in the stratum corneum, the topmost layer of the skin, they plump up those cells. As a result, skin becomes softer and smoother and fine lines are less noticeable.

Other anti-aging products are treatments that promote "cell renewal." These contain ingredients that speed the rate at which new cells are formed in the epidermis, grow, rise to the stratum corneum, and then are shed or sloughed off. When the cycle is accelerated, cells tend to be younger by the time they reach the surface, and the result can be skin that is more translucent and glowing. What is not mentioned in the ads, of course, is that the gentle friction of a washcloth, complexion brush, or granular scrub also tends to speed cell growth and exfoliation, as can the mild irritation of a chemical exfoliant. The relationship of cell renewal products to washcloth or clarifying lotion is much the same as that of the newest generation of anti-aging moisturizers to ordinary moisturizing creams and lotions. They accomplish similar ends by more advanced, (possibly) more efficient, and (certainly) more expensive means.

In 1987 the Food and Drug Administration notified several beauty companies that unless they could back up claims that their products actually change the way skin functions—in which case, those products would need to be approved as drugs and sold by prescription—the companies would have to stop making anti-aging claims. As a result, outright anti-aging claims on labels and packaging and in ads have been replaced by subtler hints and implications.

Does this mean that new, state-of-the-art treatments are useless? Not at all. Some of the moisturizers, especially those containing hyaluronic acid, are excellent, as are a few of the "cell renewal" products made with proteins, such as glycoprotein. Just keep in mind that most are scientifically advanced variations on old themes. They won't work wonders, though some do seem to outperform ordinary moisturizers and exfoliants. Youth *still* can't be bought in a bottle, jar, or even an ampoule.

If you like the idea of using the latest fruits of the cosmetic chemists' labors and can afford these products, by all means, give them a try. Do keep the following points in mind when you make your selections.

• Know what you are getting. Descriptions in ads and on labels of some of the products under consideration often make it difficult to determine exactly what a cream, lotion, gel, et cetera, is supposed to do for you. As a general rule, though, when a label mentions smoothing, softening, rehydration, and wrinkle reduction, the product is a moisturizer. If the implied benefits are polished, fresher-looking, more translucent, or more elastic skin, it is probably a cell renewal product. (Some products combine both functions.)

• If your skin is sensitive, test any new product before using it on your face by applying some to the inside of your elbow. Smooth it on and wait a day or so to see how skin reacts. (Naturally, if the area turns red or itchy, that product is not for you.) You don't have to purchase full-size bottles or jars to test. Ask for free samples. Or use the in-store testers made available by many manufacturers.

• No matter what the salesperson might say to the contrary, it is not necessary to buy an entire line of products—including, for example, a day cream, a night cream, an eye cream, a throat cream, and so on—to get the benefits of any single one. You need only purchase what you want and need, and can mix and match different brands.

The first two categories of anti-agers—moisturizers and cell-renewal agents—go to work immediately. That doesn't mean you'll see an instant, significant difference, just that ingredients in the products begin to affect your skin soon after they're applied. The third category of products works preventively to protect against skin devastation. These products are sun blocks and sunscreens.

There's no doubt that they work. Every person, man or woman, who is the least bit concerned about good looks and good health should wear a sun protection product—not just at the beach or on the tennis court in summer, but all day, every day, year round. That's because skin is constantly exposed to sunlight and damage can occur even indoors, in a sunlit room.

What's the nature of the damage? In addition to the dryness and coarsened or leathery texture that constant exposure to the sun can lead to, sunlight inflicts injury to *fibroblasts*. These are cells that produce collagen and elastin, the fibrous proteins giving skin firmness, tone, and elasticity—the ability to snap back to its original shape after being stretched out or bunched up. When fibroblasts in the dermis are rendered less efficient by sunlight, there are qualitative and quantitative changes in collagen and elastin. As a result, skin recovers more slowly and less well when creased into a frown, smile, or other expression (even from being slept on the "wrong way" at night!), until lines gradually become permanent and deepen into furrows. Deteriorated collagen and elastin also allow the force of gravity to get the upper hand, and skin begins to sag. There's more. Among the many other changes thought to be a direct result of sun exposure are irregularities in pigmentation: increased freckling, mottling, and in late middle age, the appearance of liver spots.

To see the extent of sun damage to *your* skin, compare your face—the most exposed part of your body—with skin that is ordinarily covered (the insides of thighs, buttocks, abdomen). Though facial skin is different from skin on those other areas in that it is more plentifully supplied with oil glands, practically all the difference in color, texture, tone, and wrinkling or lack of it is due to changes caused by sunlight.

And in reviewing the aging effects of the sun, I haven't even touched on the most important problem caused by ultraviolet rays: Sun exposure is a primary risk factor in the development of skin cancer.

Though damage isn't visible to the naked eye until the age of thirty or so, electron micrography shows that sun-related changes in the skin are often well under way in early childhood. For this reason, I and many other dermatologists urge patients who are new parents to begin routine use of sun protection products on their children in infancy and to keep children indoors during the middle of the day when the sun's rays are strongest. Damage is cumulative. The more sun exposure on skin over the years, the more harm that will result. It's never too early or too late to start sheltering your skin from the sun. It's the most valuable anti-aging technique of all.

Sun Protection—What to Use, and How

As you've undoubtedly noticed, a wide variety of cosmetics and treatment products now contain ingredients that provide sun protection. Other products are sold separately as sunscreens— which act as chemical shields that prevent ultraviolet rays from penetrating through to the skin—and sun blocks, which deflect the rays, causing them to bounce harmlessly off the skin. Some are marketed for whole-body protection at the beach, the golf course, the tennis courts, and are meant to be applied to all exposed skin. Many of these are manufactured by the same companies that make tanning lotions and gels. Other products, often made by cosmetics companies, are sold as "face savers," to be worn alone or under makeup.

All have an SPF (sun protection factor) number clearly indicated on package or label. The numbers range from 2 to 50; the higher the number, the greater the protection offered by the product.

Many beauty experts and even some dermatologists suggest that the SPF of a sunscreen be related to an individual's tanning potential. According to them, if your skin is fair, your eyes blue or gray, your hair light or reddish, and if instead of tanning, you freckle and burn within minutes of going out unprotected into strong sunlight, you should use products with an SPF of 15 or more. At the other end of the spectrum, if your skin is brown or black, your eyes and hair are dark, and if you can spend long periods in the sun without burning, a product with an SPF of 2 or 4 offers enough protection. In between these two extremes are people with varying degrees of tanning potential, and each is assigned an appropriate SPF.

Unfortunately, this method of assigning a suitable SPF was developed to allow "safe" light tanning without burning. In view of what we now know about the damage ultraviolet rays can inflict, it's obvious that no tan is a safe tan and that everyone, regardless of skin color, should take advantage of the optimal protection offered by high SPF products.

My simplified recommendation with regard to sun protection is to choose and wear a product with an SPF of at least 8 if your skin is black, and 15 if your skin is brown to very fair.

The product you choose should protect against the two most damaging types of rays: UVBs, which are strongest between the hours of 10:00 A.M. and 2:00 P.M. when the sun is at its peak, and UVAs (once thought to be harmless), which bombard us at all hours of the day. UVAs are less concentrated, but penetrate more deeply into the skin and intensify the effects of UVBs. Check labels and select a product that protects against both types of rays. (Sometimes terms such as "broad-spectrum," or "full-spectrum," are used to indicate that a product screens or blocks UVBs and UVAs.)

You should also be aware of the fact that some sun protection products have an alcohol or water base and others are oil-based. Since you should be wearing a sunscreen or sun block every day, it's important to match it to your skin. Unfortunately, few products now are identified on labels as being for oily skin, or dry skin, and so on, so be sure to scan labels to find compatible sun protection.

• If your skin is oily, look for a product listing water and/or alcohol at the top of the ingredient list, followed by no or few oily ingredients, such as Sundown Sun Block 15 (Johnson & Johnson) or Supershade 15 Oil-Free, Clear Gel Sun Block. Be especially careful to avoid sun protection products containing coconut oil and cocoa butter.

• If you have combination skin, choose an alcohol or water-based product unless your cheeks and the area around your mouth are very dry. In that case, consider using two products— one listing alcohol or water and no oil among its first two or three ingredients for forehead, nose, and chin, and one listing an oil near the top of the ingredient list for areas outside the T-zone.

• If your skin is normal, select a product according to whether you are going through a dry phase (in which case you should wear one listing an oil among the first two or three ingredients), or an oily period (select sun protection with alcohol or water at the top of the ingredient list). If your skin is perfectly normal, be guided by your own preference with regard to how a product feels on your skin.

• If your skin is dry, of course, look for a product with an oil as one of the first two or three ingredients, such as Coppertone Moisturizing Sunblock Lotion or Neutrogena PABA-free sunscreen.

• If your skin is sensitive or you are allergy-prone, watch out for ingredients that might provoke a reaction. Fragrance and alcohol are among the most likely irritators of sensitive skin. PABA, a common sunscreen ingredient, sometimes produces an allergic reaction in those who are allergic to anesthetics such as benzocaine and lidocaine, or to certain hair dyes. Salicylates and cinnamates, sometimes present as octyl methoxy-cinnamate, have resulted in contact dermatitis in a few individuals. Of course, discontinue use of any product that seems to be causing problems. Then try one with a different formulation. Look for products labeled for sensitive skin, such as PreSun Sensitive Skin Sunscreen. If you're unable to find a product that doesn't upset your skin, tell your dermatologist what you have used in the past and what happened when you used it. He or she should be able to come up with some trouble-free alternatives.

There are a few other factors to consider when selecting sun protection. If you're a serious swimmer or jogger, for example, or if you frequently spend hours outdoors engaged in strenuous activity that causes you to perspire, get a waterproof product. Even these, however, need to be reapplied after swimming for more than an hour or when perspiration is heavy. Check the label to find out how often to smooth on more.

When choosing a product to wear under makeup, make sure its color and texture won't interfere with cosmetics. (Some sunscreens are almost transparent, some are tinted a medium flesh tone, some are creamy white when applied but soon blend in with skin color and vanish.)

Many sun protection preparations are promoted for use on

the face, alone or under makeup. Others, the "beach products," are marketed to appeal to sunbathers and sports enthusiasts who want allover protection. Keep in mind that you may not need two sunscreens, one for your face and one for your body. The right product, one with a high SPF and which satisfies other requirements mentioned above, can be used on face *and* body. The exception of course is when facial skin is oily and body skin is dry. In that case, you'll need one with a water base for your face and another, with moisturizing ingredients, for your body.

How to Get Maximum Sun Protection

The suggestions that follow should help you obtain optimal benefits from a sunscreen or sun block. However, don't neglect to read the manufacturer's instructions and adhere to them if they conflict with any of the guidelines below.

• Whenever possible, apply sunscreen or sun block an hour before you go out of doors.
• To shield your face, apply the product after moisturizer but before makeup. You can, if you wish, use a sunscreen with built-in moisturizing ingredients in place of an ordinary moisturizer.
• Be sure to use enough of the product for complete coverage. Don't massage it into your skin. Smooth it on without rubbing, using overlapping strokes so there won't be any gaps in protection.
• Apply the product to all exposed areas of your body, including your hands. (They're just as vulnerable to aging rays—and show it just as quickly—as your face.)

There's no way to know exactly what your skin will be like years from now if you start protecting it from the sun today. But it will certainly be healthier and younger looking than if you didn't.

Age Erasers

Sun protection is skin insurance for the future. The techniques that follow can give you a more youthful look right now.

Special-Occasion Facial

The facial described below helps brighten skin, plump out fine lines, and subtract years, for a few hours anyway. Since it takes about sixty minutes from start to finish, it's not for everyday. Save it for when you want to look your best.

NOTE: Because the ingredients for this facial include prod-ucts containing oil, and physical exfoliants, don't use it when your skin is blemished or if you are acne-prone. If your skin is clear but sensitive, step 5—rubbing it with sugar—might be too irritating. Use baking soda instead, or omit step 5 completely.

Gather a light oil, such as baby oil; your usual cleanser and toner; sugar (or baking soda); a moisturizer (preferably one that contains urea, hyaluronic acid, glycerin, or other humec-tants); two old, clean washcloths; a bowl containing ice cubes and water. A few hours before you begin, place toner in the refrigerator so that it will be well-chilled when you use it.

1. In the top part of a double boiler, place a measuring cup containing two to three tablespoons of moisturizer. Fill the bot-tom part of the double boiler halfway with water and set on the stove over very low heat. When the moisturizer is liquefied, remove it from the heat.

2. Tie back your hair and clean away makeup with cotton balls dampened with light oil.

3. Cleanse your face as usual. Rinse with warm water. Do not use toner or moisturizer.

4. Pour several drops of oil into the palm of your hand. Rub palms together to distribute the oil, then stroke it onto your face.

5. Pour several more drops of oil into palm, add about a

teaspoon of sugar and stroke it *lightly* over your face. Then, using the balls of your fingers only, and exerting the gentlest possible pressure, massage in smallish circles. Do not rub. Do not overwork any one area. Avoid upper and lower lids and the tender skin just below your eyes. Stop after one minute.

6. Rinse your face thoroughly with warm running water.

7. Blot with a clean towel until your face is almost but not quite dry.

8. Test the temperature of liquefied moisturizer. It should be warm but not hot. (If it's hot, wait until it's cool enough to feel comfortable when you rub some on the inside of your wrist.) Apply generously to your face. Saturate washcloths with warm water, then wring them out. Lie down and arrange the cloths vertically on your face so that each covers half, leaving room for breathing.

9. Rest for ten minutes. Saturate cloths again in warm water, wring them out and arrange on your face as before, then lie down and rest for another ten minutes.

10. Rinse by splashing several times with warm water. Gradually adjust temperature to cold. Dip a washcloth in ice water, wring it out, and press it against your face for thirty seconds or so.

11. Blot your face damp-dry, apply chilled toner with cotton balls, smooth on a thin film of moisturizer (this time from the jar). And that's it. Your face is refreshed, toned, ready for makeup.

Heavy-Duty Remedies for Wrinkles

Many patients tell me they don't mind their wrinkles. And I believe them. But many more *do* mind them. (Some of these don't seem to care a bit about getting older; it's *looking* older that bothers them.) They mind so much they're willing to undergo minor physical discomfort and financial expense in order to get rid of their wrinkles. It *can* be done. But you can't buy the supplies and equipment for heavy-duty wrinkle fixing on your own. To get the benefits of collagen, Retin-A, chemical peels, and other wrinkle fixes, you need the help of a dermatologist or other doctor.

How do these procedures work, and are they for you? Those are the questions I'll be answering in this section.

Collagen

Several times in this book I've mentioned collagen, the fibrous protein, produced in the dermis, which provides much of the underlying support structure of the skin. In young skin, collagen fibers are plentiful and intact. Over the years, the stress of sun exposure, smiling, frowning, squinting, et cetera, the tug of gravity, and for some, infection, illness, poor eating habits (particularly deprivation dieting), along with other factors, promote the breakdown of the once-firm and springy network of collagen fibers. At the same time, bone and muscle mass, and subcutaneous facial fat decrease. Skin no longer fits properly. The excess folds into tiny lines, wrinkles, creases, furrows.

For many years, researchers experimented with various substances that could be injected into the skin to smooth out lines and fill in furrows and other depressions. Injectible collagen, formulated with bovine collagen similar to our own, and first used on patients in 1976, proved to be effective.

How does it work? Small amounts of collagen are injected into the dermis to replace lost tissue. The material then functions as a framework into which new skin cells can grow; in supplementing the body's own collagen, wrinkled areas are recontoured. In most cases the corrections are completed in two to four sessions, usually spaced two weeks apart; each session takes fifteen to thirty minutes. Zyderm Collagen I and II can be used to fill in shallow forehead lines, crow's feet, "laugh lines" running from sides of nose to mouth, vertical lines above and below the lips, and certain types of scars. Zyplast Collagen, newer and stronger than Zyderm I and II, effectively fills in deeper furrows and scars. Unfortunately, none are very good for rais-ing depressed scars with sharp edges, such as the "ice pick" scars that are an aftermath of some cases of acne.

Some of my patients say the injections, made with a very fine-gauge needle, feel like a pinch or twinge (one woman com-pared it to the fleeting sting of having an eyebrow tweezed). Lidocaine, a mild anesthetic, is mixed into the collagen, and as a result, when a small area is injected more than once, the second and third injections are felt less keenly than the first. After treatment, there is almost always some redness and swell-ing, which usually subsides by the following day. However, I have had more than one patient who, after receiving colla-gen injections in the afternoon, went out to a party—in full makeup—that very same evening.

Is it permanent? No. Injectible collagen is subject to the same forces that cause breakdown and deterioration of the body's own collagen. Recontouring tends to last anywhere from six to eighteen months, depending on a variety of factors, such as the amount of stress in the area (how often and how vigorously facial muscles are used, for example), and the patient's body chemistry. After that, periodic touch-up injections are needed to maintain the original corrections. According to research done by the Collagen Corporation, makers of Zyderm and Zy-plast, most patients who return for touch-ups do so within six months to a year of the initial series. Touch-ups, incidentally, are often just that, usually requiring less collagen and fewer sessions than the first time around.

Is it for you? Yes, if a skin test, given four weeks before, indi-cates that you are not sensitive to the material. Approximately 3 percent of potential patients prove allergic to collagen and cannot proceed with treatment. Slightly more than 1 percent of treated patients develop hypersensitivity—greater than usual redness and swelling at the injection site—despite negative test results. Fortunately, such reactions, when they occur, resolve themselves without treatment.

Yes, if you can afford it. Fees vary depending on the extent of the corrections and the area involved. A series of treatments might cost as little as $400 to $800, but could be considerably more. Insurance companies often reimburse for correction of scarring resulting from injury or acne, but not for purely cosmetic treatment.

Yes, if your expectations are realistic. If you're unhappy about frown lines on your forehead, puckered skin around your mouth, or crow's feet, collagen treatments can solve your problems. Collagen is not a cure for jowls, undereye bags, or puffy upper lids. For those and other problems involving excess skin, plastic surgery is the only answer.

Retin-A

Earlier in this chapter, the aging effects of ultraviolet rays, and how to prevent photoaging, were discussed. What's the difference between photoaging and ordinary biological aging? Not a great deal, at least in terms of the way skin looks to the naked eye. A consensus seems to be developing among researchers that photoaging and biological aging are hard to differentiate, and that whatever the factors that cause biological aging, the process is accelerated by sun exposure. Retin-A, a synthetic vitamin A derivative marketed in cream and gel form by Ortho Pharmaceutical, appears to reverse many of the signs of photoaging.

How does it work? Actually, we don't yet know *why* Retin-A causes certain cellular changes in the stratum corneum, epidermis, and dermis, but we have a good idea of *how* skin responds to Retin-A applied regularly over a period of months.

For one thing, there is accelerated shedding of dead skin cells from the stratum corneum, which then becomes smoother, thinner, and as a result reflects light more evenly—much as young skin does.

In addition, new cells seem to be generated more quickly and rise more rapidly from the epidermis to the stratum corneum so that the latter is made up, literally, of younger cells. These cells are less prone to the clumping that can make older skin feel and look rough or leathery.

As the stratum corneum thins, the epidermis—which becomes thinner with advancing years and sun exposure—begins to thicken up again. It may be this epidermal thickening that accounts for the smoothing out of fine lines and wrinkles noticed by so many users of Retin-A and well-documented by ordinary photographs and electron micrography.

Retin-A also appears to encourage development of blood vessels and capillaries that supply oxygen and nourishment to skin cells. With an increased supply of blood, skin often loses the sallow, faded appearance of age and takes on a more youthful rosiness.

Retin-A tends to fade out freckles and age spots, sometimes causing them to disappear completely.

Most important from a health standpoint is that Retin-A can inhibit the development of precancerous lesions, and perhaps prevent certain types of skin cancers.

What's the downside? Retin-A, to be effective, must be used frequently, regularly (some dermatologists suggest nightly application for some patients, and every-other-night use for others), and carefully. The regimen includes gentle cleansing in the evening, followed by a twenty- to thirty-minute wait, after which a very small amount of Retin-A is smoothed on. In the morning, skin is cleansed again. After that, a moisturizer and sunscreen are applied.

In my opinion, reports in the media about extreme irritation, dryness, and flakiness as a result of using Retin-A have been exaggerated. Certainly the potential for irritation is there. However, I've found that problems are rare when a patient is started on a mild formulation (the product is available in several strengths), uses it in small amounts, and follows my instructions to cleanse very gently with a mild soap such as Purpose or a soap substitute (I prefer SFC Lotion for my Retin-A patients).

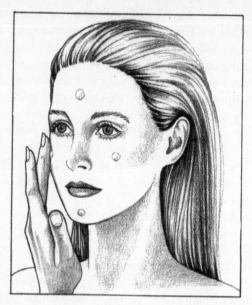

For best results, Retin-A should be dotted on sparingly, as shown. Smooth it in, avoiding corners of eyes, mouth, and the area immediately surrounding nostrils.

With continued use, initial minor irritation, if any, usually subsides and skin soon returns to normal, only better. Optimal results seem to be achieved within a year, after which the patient may choose to maintain the improvements with weekly or twice-weekly applications of Retin-A.

A drawback potentially more serious than minor irritation has to do with the fact that as Retin-A thins the stratum corneum, the skin becomes more vulnerable and sensitive to the sun than before. Researchers are now attempting to evaluate the long-term implications of increased sun sensitivity. In the meantime, it is *absolutely essential* for anyone using Retin-A to wear broad-spectrum sun protection with an SPF of 15 or higher all day, every day.

Is it for you? Yes, if your skin can tolerate regular, frequent application of the preparation. As I noted earlier, when

Retin-A is properly used, irritation tends to be minor, except for those individuals who have extremely sensitive skin.

Yes, if you know you can be diligent about using sun protection products. Even after you have used Retin-A for a year and are on once-a-week maintenance, sunscreening remains a must.

Yes, if you can afford the relatively small expense of an initial visit to a doctor, plus periodic follow-up appointments that might be necessary to adjust the concentration or format of the product to better suit your skin, and to assess progress. There is also the cost of the Retin-A itself—approximately $25 for a three-month supply.

Yes, if you're prepared to wait for results. Improvement is often so slow and gradual, it goes unnoticed until one day, perhaps three, four, five months after you start to use it, you recognize that, yes, your skin *is* smoother, clearer, less wrinkled. Retin-A won't suddenly make you over into a ravishing twenty-three-year-old if you're pushing fifty. All it will do is make your skin look better and younger. But that's a lot, isn't it?

Chemical Peels

Chemical peels remove the outer skin layers—and fine lines and wrinkles along with them. Whereas collagen and Retin-A therapy are in a sense lunch-hour treatments—which, except for the time you spend in your doctor's office, don't interrupt your life—a chemical peel almost always requires some rescheduling. Though a full-face peel takes about an hour, and peeling smaller areas fifteen to thirty minutes, you will probably want to avoid appearing in public for at least a week and possibly ten days afterward. However, results tend to be long lasting. Wrinkles removed by a peel are gone or lessened. And though new wrinkles might develop, it could be five, ten, even twenty years before they become significant.

How does it work? Peels are often administered on an outpatient basis in a doctor's office, or in a hospital operating room. (In some cases, patients are encouraged to spend the night following the procedure in the hospital.) Chemicals of various strengths—often trichloracetic acid or buffered phenol—are swabbed over the entire face or on selected areas, such as near the corners of the eyes to remove crow's feet, or around the mouth to get rid of vertical lines radiating from upper and lower lips. The chemical solution is left on for about a minute, then treated areas may be taped.

Three days after the procedure, the patient returns to the doctor's office for a progress check and to have the tape removed. Thymol iodide powder may be applied to dry oozing and help prevent infection. Skin is dark pink or red at this point. Throbbing and swelling are common, but discomfort may be eased by sitting or standing instead of resting in bed.

Crusting, which can form over peeled areas, is often minimized by frequent splashing with tepid water. It's important not to attempt to remove crusts without first checking with the doctor on the proper way to do so.

Significant redness and swelling last about eight to ten days following the treatment. (A not unattractive pinkness may linger on for six weeks.) Between ten and fourteen days after the peel cosmetics can be used. Though patients are back to "normal" well before, the final outcome cannot be judged for about six months, when *all* swelling has subsided. That's because even a slightly swollen face tends to look smoother and less wrinkled than it really is.

What about side effects and complications? New skin formed after a peel is always a somewhat different color than the old skin that was removed. A person with freckles will be freckle-free in peeled areas, but not elsewhere. Pores may be temporarily enlarged, and moles darker. There is a small chance of scarring, especially in people who tend to develop thick scar tissue over a wound. (Estimates are that 5 to 10 percent of chemical peel patients scar as a result of the procedure; in most cases, though, scarring gradually fades to near invisibility.

It is extremely important to avoid exposure to direct and indirect or reflected sunlight for several weeks after the tapes have been removed. In some instances, even a few seconds of exposure has altered pigmentation enough to affect the final results. Still more important is the fact that when upper skin cell layers are removed, tanning is no longer possible. But burning is. This means that chemical peel patients put themselves at greater risk for developing skin cancers unless they commit themselves to a lifetime of using broad-spectrum, high SPF sun protection.

Is it for you? Yes, if your skin is fair to medium in color—the kind of skin that tends to wrinkle more, and earlier, than darker skin. Olive, brown, black, and especially Asian skin can become severely blotched, sometimes permanently, by chemical peels. In fact, most reputable doctors will refuse to perform the procedure if there is any likelihood that major pigmentation irregularities will result.

Yes, if you are in good physical health, with no apparent heart trouble. Small amounts of phenol, one of the chemicals often used in peeling, enter the bloodstream during the treatment and can irritate the heart. When the heart is sound, this is ordinarily no problem. But it could be dangerous for those who have arrhythmias or other heart conditions.

Yes, if you understand that there will be some pain (your doctor will, of course, prescribe something to minimize discomfort), and that there is a small but real possibility that because of pigment changes, scarring, or accidental sun exposure, your new, wrinkle-free face might be otherwise less than perfect.

Yes, if you are satisfied that you have put yourself in the hands of a skilled doctor who is experienced in the procedure, and who believes the chances of obtaining the desired results are good.

Yes, if you can accept the fact that you must wear a sunscreen or sun block every day and that peeled areas will never again take a tan.

Yes, if you can afford the cost of the procedure: around $1,000 for a partial peel done in a doctor's office, up to $2,500 or more for a full peel performed in-office or at a hospital and involving an overnight stay.

Other Wrinkle-Fixing Options

Other wrinkle-removing procedures less frequently used and less well known than the big three just discussed include liquid silicone injections, "fat transfer," dermabrasion, and Fibrel. Each, when administered by a skilled doctor with experience in the procedure, can be a powerful weapon in the battle against signs of aging.

Liquid silicone. This material is not approved by the FDA for sale in the United States, yet many American doctors buy it elsewhere and use it routinely for smoothing shallow to deep wrinkles and for recontouring facial depressions. With a fine-gauge needle, the material is injected, droplet by droplet, into the skin, where it appears to stimulate production of more collagen. Silicone treatment is permanent, which is both an advantage and a disadvantage. On the plus side, once treatment is completed, it never has to be repeated. On the minus side, overcorrecting—injecting too much, or injecting it into areas where it may not be needed—does happen, though rarely, when a doctor lacks experience with the material. In addition, when administered by unskilled hands, liquid silicone can migrate; what was initially injected into a forehead line could eventually travel to the eye area, or elsewhere, for example. However, when tiny amounts of silicone are injected over a period of several months by an experienced doctor who is skilled in the procedure, chances of overcorrection and migration are greatly reduced.

Fat transfer. In this procedure, more properly called microlipo injections, some of the patient's own fat is "vacuumed" from one part of the body, placed in a syringe, and injected into deep furrows, scars, and areas that have become hollowed or sunken with age (such as the cheeks) or deformed by physical trauma. The two-step procedure—"harvesting" the fat and then injecting it where it is needed—is more complicated and time consuming for patient and doctor than simple collagen injections, and there is some risk of infection. But there's no chance of the body reacting negatively to its own fat, and there is a virtually unlimited supply of the material (even relatively thin patients have enough fat to correct and/or recontour large areas). The large-gauge needle, which must be used to deliver the fat, represents a potential drawback, since in inexperienced hands it does not lend itself to precision either in terms of exact placement or quantity of fat delivered. And, because of the size of the needle, there may be minor scarring at the point of injection. The technique is still quite new and will undoubtedly be refined. Even now, though, many doctors are enthusiastic about this procedure, which allows them to correct deeper, larger areas and offers long-lasting results, without the side effects of adverse skin reactions, such as irritation and allergy.

Autologous lipo-collagen transplantation. A new procedure pioneered in Europe, "auto-col" (for short), is a method for filling in lines, furrows, and depressions that offers many of the benefits of injectible collagen and fat transfer, without their primary drawbacks. In this procedure, performed in a doctor's office, a small amount of the patient's own fat is removed with a syringe. (In women, it's usually taken from the inner thigh or the fatty pad on the inner knee.) The fat is mixed with distilled water, which makes it nonviable but does not affect the septae—a fibrous substance in the fat containing collagen. After areas to be filled in are numbed with ice, the solution is injected. The body does not react negatively to its own collagen (remember, a small percentage of patients are sensitive to injectible bovine collagen), and because fine-gauge needles are used, corrections can be more precise and there is less chance of scarring than in fat transfer. The supply of fat-containing collagen is virtually unlimited, and more fat than is required for one session can be removed, frozen, and stored for subsequent sessions. This should translate into lower cost for the patient. The procedure is so new, we don't know how long auto-col corrections last, but the duration appears to compare favorably with that of injectible collagen.

Dermabrasion. Like chemical peeling, dermabrasion removes upper skin layers. It's performed with a high-speed mechanical abrader fitted with a stainless steel wire brush or diamond-surfaced wheel that rubs skin off in much the same way that wood is sanded. The procedure removes more skin than chemical peeling—more, in fact, than is necessary for removing fine lines and wrinkles. For this reason, dermabrasion is best reserved for smoothing and evening out deeper creases and lines, and for correcting the deep, sharp-edged scars that are the aftermath of some severe cases of acne.

Fibrel. Approved by the FDA in mid-1988 for use in the correction of scarring, Fibrel is also showing great promise as a wrinkle fixer. The material is composed of the patient's own blood, a gelatin powder, and a clotting agent. When injected into the skin, the mixture encourages new, natural collagen to form at the site; over a period of two to four months, the material is entirely replaced by natural collagen. The procedure, which involves drawing blood from the patient and mixing it with other ingredients, is more complicated than collagen injections, but because Fibrel is less allergenic, it often works for people who cannot tolerate injectible collagen. In addition, Fibrel corrections tend to be longer-lasting, though some patients return for touch-up treatments after a year. Like collagen, Fibrel is delivered with a very fine-gauge needle that can be used with great precision, and rarely, if ever, leaves scars. In experienced hands, and administered to the right patient—one who doesn't expect miracles, just good results—Fibrel is an excellent stop-the-clock treatment.

Anti-aging treatments don't stop here, of course. For the woman or man who is highly motivated to maintain youthful contours

and is willing to bear the cost in dollars, time, discomfort—
and possibly some pain—there is an ever-widening range of
cosmetic surgical procedures that are beyond the scope of this
book. I'm talking now about face lifts, brow lifts, cheek and
chin implants, surgery to firm up upper and lower eyelids ...
the list could go on and on. There are several good books on
the subject, most of them written by cosmetic plastic surgeons.
One of the best is *The Complete Book of Plastic Surgery*, by Elizabeth Morgan, M.D., F.A.C.S., published by Warner Books, New
York, 1988. If you are contemplating a face lift or other plastic
procedure, these books will advise you about costs, how various
procedures are performed, what kind of results to expect, how
to take care of yourself after surgery, and so on.

But, some people wonder, what's the point of spending so
much time, money, and energy on efforts to look younger?
Why not just grow old gracefully? Why not indeed? If main-
taining a youthful appearance seems like a waste, then it certainly is, for those who feel that way. But it seems to me that
for the rest of us, looking young is not really the goal. It's
looking *good*—and the heightened self-confidence that comes
from knowing we're at our best.

Do you have a question or comment about your skin? Dr. Haberman will be happy to answer it. Write to him at the address below.
(To speed things along, put the words "Beauty Hotline" on the
envelope.) Enclose a self-addressed, stamped, business-size envelope with your query.

Dr. Fredric Haberman, Medical Director
Affiliated Dermatology and Plastic Surgery Center
19-21 Fairlawn Avenue
Fair Lawn, NJ 07410

Index